ELTING MEMORIAL LIBRARY NEW PALTZ

D0204249

MAXIMIZING YOUR HEALTH INSURANCE BENEFITS

A Consumer's Guide to New and Traditional Plans

RICHARD EPSTEIN

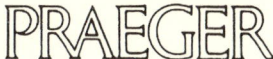

Westport, Connecticut
London

Library of Congress Cataloging-in-Publication Data

Epstein, Richard, 1939–
    Maximizing your health insurance benefits : a consumer's guide to
new and traditional plans / Richard Epstein.
      p. cm.
    Includes bibliographical references and index.
    ISBN 0–275–95510–9 (alk. paper)
    1. Insurance, Health—United States. 2. Consumer education—
Handbooks, manuals, etc. I. Title.
    HG9396.E67 1997
    368.38′2′00297—dc21   97–8861

British Library Cataloguing in Publication Data is available.

Library of Congress Catalog Card Number: 97–8861
ISBN: 0–275–95510–9

First published in 1997

Praeger Publishers, 88 Post Road West, Westport, CT 06881
An imprint of Greenwood Publishing Group, Inc.

Printed in the United States of America

The paper used in this book complies with the
Permanent Paper Standard issued by the National
Information Standards Organization (Z39.48–1984).

10 9 8 7 6 5 4 3 2 1

For my wife, Carolyn, whose enormous patience and superb editing skills have helped to make this book possible, and for my children, Jay, Joanna, and Eric.

Contents

Tables

Acknowledgments

A number of individuals have been particularly helpful in the preparation of this book. Several people have helped to edit the book, so that it's easy for readers to use and understand. A number of other individuals have contributed specific factual information, or have helped me to understand the technicalities of specific laws and regulations.

I want to thank Herb Jurist and Jeffrey Kassover, who patiently read the book and made a variety of helpful suggestions. In terms of technical advice and information, I particularly want to thank the following people (listed in alphabetical order)

- Diane Archer and Judy Ng (Medicare Rights Center);
- Julie Beckett (National Coordinator, Family Voices);
- Kevin Brown, Chief Master Sergeant (Senior Enlisted Representative for CHAMPUS);
- Richard Coorsh, Harvie Raymond, and Tom O'Hare (Health Insurance Association of America);
- Lauren Ewers (Health Policy Fellow to Senator Edward M. Kennedy, United States Senate Committee on Labor and Human Resources);
- Mark Gordon (Thomas Edison State College);
- Stanley Klein (Co-founder and Editor-in-Chief, *Exceptional Parent Magazine*);

- Susan Marquis (one of several authors of "Self-Insured Employer Health Plans: Prevalence, Profile, Provisions, and Premiums," in *Health Affairs,* Volume 15, Number 2);
- Lynne Meyer (Medical Business Associates);
- Charles Mondin, Anne Werner, Priscilla Itscoitz (United Seniors Health Cooperative);
- Sharon Morrissey and John Miller (Pension and Welfare Benefits Administration of the United States Department of Labor);
- Anne Rufo (Legislative Fellow for Senator Nancy Kassebaum, United States Senate Committee on Labor and Human Resources);
- Ken Scholen (National Center for Home Equity Conversion);
- Harry Simon, Leslie Daniels (National Health Law Program);
- Sally Tanenbaum (Executive Director, United Association for Handicapped Citizens);
- Donald White (American Association of Health Plans).

I also want to thank the many readers of my weekly newspaper column and my column in *Exceptional Parent Magazine,* whose search for solutions to their own health insurance problems has helped me to understand both the difficulties inherent in the current American system of health insurance and the need for this book. In addition, I especially want to thank Joseph Valenzano, Jr., President and Publisher of *Exceptional Parent Magazine,* for his support, encouragement, and expert advice.

Introduction

I've been writing a newspaper and magazine column on health insurance issues for a number of years. During that time, I've found that many types of health insurance problems have become rather commonplace in America. In fact, if you've been covered by a health insurance policy for more than a few years, you've probably encountered at least some of these problems

- You file a claim and never hear from your insurance company again;
- You file a claim, and your insurance company responds with a message that's so cryptic that you feel as if you need a translator to even begin to understand it;
- Your insurance company sends you a check for far less than you think you're entitled to under the terms of your policy, and you have no idea why;
- Your insurance company sends you a check for far more than you think you're entitled to under the terms of your policy, and you have no idea why;
- Your insurer sends you a letter asking you to send your claim to your automobile insurance company first, and to include a copy of the accident report when you re-file your claim, but you haven't been involved in an accident and you haven't filed a claim in months;
- Your insurance company pays your hospital bill, but then

insists that the hospital return the money, and the hospital has now asked you to pay the bill;

- You receive a check from your insurance company, but you are certain that you haven't filed a claim;
- You've been reimbursed twice by your insurance company for the same claim;
- You've had the same insurance policy with the same company for years, but your insurer has suddenly begun to reject your claims on the grounds that you've never been insured with the company;
- Your Medicare carrier has informed you that Medicare is now your secondary insurer, and that your primary insurer is a company you've never heard of;
- Your insurer insists that your doctor's bill is far above the usual and customary rate, but your doctor assures you that her fees are the same as, or lower than, other doctors in the area;
- Your insurance company has requested additional information before it will continue processing your claim, but no one to whom you've spoken at the insurance company seems to be certain what information is required.

I've found that a large percentage of such problems, including many of those that seem overwhelmingly complex at first, turn out to be the result of either simple claim-processing errors or difficulties in communication. Once the nature of the problem becomes clear, it's often fairly easy to find a solution.

However, in order to analyze a health insurance problem, you need to have the proper tools. That's true of almost all fields. Whether you're trying to build a new deck on your house, repair your car, or make sense of your taxes, you need to have the right tools in order to do the job properly. This book is designed to help you develop the tools you need to solve your health insurance problems. I hope, as well, that the book will allow for the development of an overall understanding of the current health insurance system in America, so that you can participate more effectively in the current debate on health care and health insurance reform.

This book is intended to meet the needs of a number of specific groups, including

- consumers insured through individual health insurance policies, employment-based group health insurance plans, HMOs or other types of managed care plans, self-funded plans, or CHAMPUS;
- individuals covered by Medicare, Medigap policies or secondary health insurance policies, or Medicare HMOs;
- children and adults with disabilities or special health care needs who are covered by Medicaid or by private health insurance policies;
- parents of children with disabilities or special health care needs who are seeking an alternate method of paying for medical expenses;
- people trying to help a friend or relative deal with a health insurance problem;
- people who are trying to help their parents or grandparents obtain coverage for home health care, nursing home care, or other types of long-term care;
- professionals such as doctors, nurses, benefits managers, human resource managers, claims supervisors, and hospital billing department supervisors.

THE STRUCTURE OF THIS BOOK

In order to make this book as easy as possible to use and to understand, I've written it with a focus on practical concerns—a "how to" approach—rather than on theoretical or statistical issues. Thus, many theoretical issues have been discussed only in general terms rather than in detail.

Technical terminology has been kept to a minimum, and only those terms that are regularly used in the health insurance field to communicate with consumers have been included. In addition, each technical term has been printed in bold print the first time it appears in the book. Complex terms are illustrated by examples, and each term is followed by an explanation.

To allow readers to learn how to deal with health insurance problems as quickly as possible, I've divided the book into four separate parts. Each part deals with a different issue, and each of the chapters within a particular part has its own focus.

Part I, "The Basic Tools," presents an overview of the current health insurance system. It deals with the technical language of health insurance and with ways to help prevent health insurance claim problems from occurring. In addition, it shows readers how to develop a system to deal with problems that do occur. Part II, "Health Insurance Plans," offers a detailed discussion of traditional individual and group health insurance plans, self-funded plans, HMOs and other types of managed care plans, Medical Savings Accounts, and other health insurance programs.

Part III, "Medicare and Medicare-Related Programs," deals with Medicare, Medigap policies, secondary insurance policies, and Medicare HMOs. Part IV, "Specialized Situations," includes a discussion of mechanisms for continuing health insurance coverage through COBRA, the new Portability and Accountability Act, and conversion options. It also focuses on programs designed for children and adults with disabilities and special health care needs, and reviews issues related to coverage for home health care, nursing homes, and other types of long-term care. The Conclusion deals with the future of the health insurance system in America.

There are two appendixes, as well. They are intended to help readers find answers to specific questions and to obtain additional information and advice. Appendix A offers answers to ten frequently asked questions about health insurance. Appendix B includes a list of sources of up-to-date information about various aspects of the health insurance system and a list of organizations and agencies that can provide advice in relation to specific health insurance problems.

In addition, there are tables throughout the book that summarize basic information. A glossary follows the appendixes and lists technical terms and phrases, along with a definition for each.

While it's not necessary to read the chapters in this book in the order in which they're presented, Part I (Chapters 1, 2, and 3) serves as an introduction to technical terms and general issues. It will help you establish an effective system for dealing with claims. Thus, those chapters are particularly important. Beyond that, however, if you think that a specific chapter may not relate to your needs, you can turn to the chapters that deal with those issues that are of immediate concern and return to the other sections when the issues concern you more directly.

NOTE TO THE READER

It's important for readers to understand that state and federal laws and regulations may change or may be reinterpreted periodically and that laws and regulations differ significantly from state to state. This book is designed to serve as a general guide to dealing with health insurance problems. However, readers should contact their state Department of Insurance and the organizations listed in the appendixes for up-to-date information about health insurance issues and recent changes in laws or regulations, as well as for advice in regard to specific problems. In addition, because of the complexity and the technical nature of the existing system of laws and regulations, the complexity of the current health insurance system, and the substantial differences between health insurance policies, it's essential for readers to discuss their specific health insurance problems with an appropriate state, federal, or private agency and with an attorney before making any decisions.

GETTING IN TOUCH WITH THE AUTHOR

A book such as this that attempts to summarize enormous amounts of information about a field as complex as health insurance may overlook some important facts or some important issues. If you have comments or suggestions about this book, I'd very much like to hear from you.

Although it's not generally possible for me to reply individually to letters, I'll try to incorporate suggested changes in any future editions of this book. You can write to me at: Richard Epstein, 350 Ramapo Valley Road, Ste. 18, Oakland, New Jersey 07436.

That address is only for comments and suggestions about the book. If you have a health insurance problem, and your local newspaper carries my nationally syndicated column ("Health Insurance TroubleShooter"), you can write to me about such problems in care of your local newspaper. I'll try to respond to as many health insurance questions as possible in the column. If your local paper does not carry the column, you can ask the editor to write to Globe Syndicate, 218 South Fairfax Street, Alexandria, Virginia 22314.

Part I
THE BASIC TOOLS

1

The Health Insurance Maze

The American system of health insurance has changed dramatically over the past few decades. Our current system originated on a large scale soon after World War II, as employers began to offer health insurance coverage as an employment-based benefit for employees and their families. At that point, policies were fairly simple and were intended primarily to help cover the cost of hospital care.

Over the decades, however, as outpatient treatments, medical tests, and medical equipment became more expensive, many health insurance policies began to offer additional benefits to cover those services and treatments. As the needs of the elderly, the poor, the uninsured, and people with disabilities were recognized, the state and federal government began to sponsor health insurance programs in addition to the private health insurance system. As time went on, the development of managed care programs and self-funded plans led to the introduction of a series of new concepts.

However, instead of being reorganized at some point into a single, fully integrated system, both government-sponsored and private health insurance programs have continued to develop piecemeal, in a sort of patchwork arrangement. At this point, the American health insurance system seems to have evolved into a complex, highly fragmented, chaotic maze.

For example, the federal government currently sponsors a number of separate health insurance programs, including Medicare, Medicaid, and CHAMPUS, as well as a number of regulatory programs such as COBRA and ERISA. Each of these programs is supervised by its own separate government agency, some programs are supervised by several different agencies, and each program has its own separate system of rules and regulations.

Medicare, a federal health insurance program for senior citizens and for some people with disabilities, is supervised through **HCFA,** the federal **Health Care Financing Administration.** However, **Medicaid**—a health insurance program for people whose income is below the poverty line as well as for some people with disabilities—is operated jointly by both the states and the federal government. Thus, it is supervised by both the federal government and by a separate agency in each state. **CHAMPUS,** the **Civilian Health and Medical Program of the Uniformed Services**—a health benefit program established by the federal government for eligible family members of armed forces personnel and for retired armed forces personnel—is supervised through a special national Tri-Care Support office (see Appendix B).

COBRA—a set of federal rules designed to allow eligible individuals to extend health insurance coverage under certain conditions—was passed as part of the **Congressional Omnibus Budget Reconciliation Act,** and is supervised through both the **Pension and Welfare Benefits Administration of the United States Department of Labor** and through the **United States Public Health Service.** The Department of Labor is responsible for COBRA issues related to health insurance programs offered by private insurers. The United States Public Health Service is responsible for COBRA issues related to health insurance programs sponsored by state or municipal government agencies.

In addition to these federal programs, state governments now offer a number of health insurance programs, as well. For example, some states currently offer programs to subsidize the cost of prescription medications for the elderly and for people with disabilities, to provide medical equipment for children, and to provide low-cost health insurance for children or adults whose incomes fall below the poverty line. Each state has its own set of regulations to govern the operation of each of those programs. In many states, the regulations are implemented through the state Department of Insurance or through special state insurance boards. In other states, the state Department of Health is also involved in regulating health insurance issues.

The current private health insurance system is just as complex. There are now more than 1,500 insurance companies and managed care companies in the United States. A single insurance company may offer several types of health insurance plans, including traditional individual and group plans and individual and group managed care plans. Each type of insurance plan may have its own set of rules.

Furthermore, each plan may be subdivided into a series of different benefit provisions. For example, many traditional group health insurance plans have separate benefit provisions for hospitalization, surgery, basic benefits, major medical, durable medical equipment, and for the treatment of mental or emotional illnesses. (See Chapter 2 or the glossary for an explanation of each of these terms.)

Each of those benefit provisions may follow separate rules, and each benefit provision may have a different deductible. Each of the traditional individual and group health insurance plans is also subject to laws and regulations passed by both the federal government and by the various states in which the plan operates.

However, self-funded plans—plans sponsored by a corporation, an association, a union, or a state or municipal government agency—are generally exempt from state regulations related to benefits. Instead, such plans are governed by rules established by **ERISA** (the federal **Employee Retirement Income Security Act**), a federal law, and are regulated through the Pension and Welfare Benefits Administration of the United States Department of Labor.

At this point, there are so many government-sponsored programs, private health insurance plans, and insurance-related laws and regulations on both the state and federal level, that the current health insurance maze is almost impenetrable. Just trying to identify the existing programs, the laws and regulations under which they are governed, and the agencies in charge of designing and implementing those regulations can be a challenge (See Table 1).

To make matters even more confusing, a number of health insurance companies seem to have recently begun a process of mergers, purchases, and subcontracting of benefits that's become so extensive that in some cases it's difficult to figure out who the insurer or administrator of a health insurance plan really is. I recently called a health insurance company, for example, to determine why a claim for physical therapy had not been paid. I discovered that claim-related decisions were being handled by a new company, formed as a result of a recent merger.

I called the new company, only to be informed that claims for physical therapy had been subcontracted to a separate company. When I called that company a few weeks later, I was informed that the company had just been purchased by a larger company and that all inquiries about policy now needed to be directed to that new company.

The health insurance maze is difficult enough for professionals to deal with. However, what makes the situation worse is that the current system of health insurance claim-filing and claim-processing involves the consumer directly. And unlike professionals, consumers have no training in claim-filing or claim-processing.

At this point, in addition to filling out forms for a primary insurer, photocopying bills, mailing claims, filling out secondary insurance forms, and keeping records, consumers often have to deal directly with claim-processing problems. For example, when a claim is denied, a consumer generally needs to try to figure out why the claim denial occurred. That's often difficult, since insurers are not always specific as to the reasons for a claim denial.

Table 1
Health Insurance Programs and Regulatory Agencies

Program/Agency	Description
Medicare	Federal program designed to provide health insurance for the elderly and for some people under age 65 with disabilities
Medicaid	Joint federal/state program designed to provide health insurance coverage for people whose incomes fall below the poverty line and for some people with disabilities
COBRA (Congressional Omnibus Budget Reconciliation Act)	Federal law that governs the continuation of health insurance coverage for eligible individuals
ERISA (Employee Retirement Income Security Act)	Federal law that regulates the operation of self-funded plans
CHAMPUS (Civilian Health And Medical Program of the Uniformed Services)	Federal health insurance program for eligible retired armed forces personnel and for eligible family members
Self-Funded Plans	Plans sponsored by a corporation, an association, a union, or a state or municipal government agency
HCFA (Health Care Financing Administration)	Regulates the operation of Medicare

Table 1 (Continued)

Program/Agency	Description
Private Health Insurance Companies	There are more than 1,500 health insurance companies and managed care companies in the United States at present; a single company may offer several types of health insurance plans
Pension and Welfare Benefits Administration of the United States Department of Labor	Regulates self-funded plans; also regulates COBRA rules in relation to private health insurance plans
United States Public Health Service	Regulates COBRA rules in relation to health insurance plans sponsored by state or municipal government agencies
State Departments of Insurance, state Departments of Health, special state insurance boards	Regulate private health insurance programs, hospital-related health insurance issues, and state-sponsored health insurance programs
State Health Insurance Programs	Health insurance programs designed to help senior citizens or people with disabilities purchase medications or medical equipment, or to provide low-cost health insurance to individuals whose incomes fall below the poverty line

Determining why a claim has been denied frequently involves calling the insurer, the doctor, or the hospital, and reviewing the policy provisions that relate to the claim. In some cases, claims are denied because the insurer requires a particular piece of information or paperwork—**documentation**—before the claim can be processed further.

Once the required documentation has been identified, the consumer needs to contact the doctor, testing center, or hospital to try to obtain the appropriate written material. That may involve asking the hospital or testing center for an itemized bill, or asking the doctor for a letter explaining why a particular treatment or service was medically necessary.

After the material has been obtained, the current system generally requires the consumer to send in a claim appeal, asking the insurer to review the claim once more. The documentation has to be photocopied by the consumer and sent in with the appeal. If the appeal is rejected, the system places the responsibility for filing additional appeals on the consumer, not on the insurer or the doctor.

Although such appeals—and the paperwork and record keeping that are part of the process—may eventually result in a successful resolution of claim problems in many cases, a great deal of knowledge, time, and energy are required on the part of the consumer. In addition, the whole process is often enormously frustrating.

However, many experts are convinced that there is no need for the consumer to be directly involved in routine claim-filing and claim-processing at all at this point. In fact, some experts have concluded that the present system could be completely restructured so that it's based on a computerized, electronic approach. Such a system could be set up so that routine claim-processing problems would be resolved between insurers and providers—doctors, hospitals, and testing centers—without the need for intervention by consumers. A computerized, electronic system could also completely eliminate the need for consumers to fill out and file claim forms, to photocopy bills, or to maintain detailed records. In addition, the development of a computerized, electronic claim-filing system could speed the entire process and reduce the number of claim errors. It would also be far more efficient, and could save billions of dollars.

According to a study by Thomas Edison College and the New Jersey Institute of Technology, the basis for the development of an efficient computerized, electronic claim-filing and processing system already exists (See Appendix B). Many doctors' offices, hospitals, pharmacies, and insurance companies are already computerized, and a variety of electronic recording systems—charge cards, debit cards, and electronic cards that can store vast amounts of information—are currently available.

Similar types of computerized, electronic systems are already in place in other fields. For example, you can now pay by credit card for food or clothing in almost any large store or supermarket in the United States without filling out complicated forms or answering personal questions, and without waiting hours or days for approval. In fact, the process generally requires only a few moments. You can go to any bank's automated teller machine, as well, insert your electronic card, and withdraw cash in just a few seconds.

In contrast, when you go to a doctor, a hospital, or a medical testing center you may have to present your health insurance identification card, answer complicated questions about your insurance policy, and provide the insurance company's address, your identification number, and personal medical information. In addition, you must fill out and sign a variety of forms.

When you get home, you may need to fill out claim forms, photocopy the medical bill, mail the forms, and record information about the doctor's visit so that you can make certain that the claim is processed properly. You then have to wait several weeks for a response from your insurer. If you're covered by a secondary insurance policy, you'll have to photocopy the Explanation of Benefits Statement from your primary insurer and the bill from the doctor, send those to the secondary insurer, and wait another few weeks for the secondary insurer to process the claim.

Since billions of health insurance claims are filed in the United States, that process is repeated over and over again. The amount of paper used in the current system of health insurance claim-filing and processing, and the amount of time involved for consumers, medical professionals, and insurers is almost incalculable.

Once a computerized, electronic claim-filing and claim-processing system is established, a consumer could simply present his electronic card to the doctor or hospital whenever treatment is provided. The information could then be scanned into a computer, and the claim could be automatically filed electronically. Payment could be made electronically, as well. A comparison of the systems makes the benefits of an electronic system obvious (See Table 2).

Studies are now being conducted by both private insurers and government agencies on the question of whether a computerized, electronic claim-filing and claim-processing system should be established in the United States. Given the enormous potential benefits that the development of such a system could offer, perhaps those studies should be made a national priority.

In the meantime, the health insurance system and the regulations under which it operates seem to grow more complex each year. A great deal of that complexity could probably be eliminated fairly easily. That's unlikely to occur in the immediate future, however, since Americans seem to be caught in a continuing philosophical debate about health care and health insurance.

The main issue in that debate revolves around the question of whether health insurance problems are best solved by government regulation or by the free market system. Instead of making a choice between these two approaches—each of which, I think, could work effectively, if properly designed and administered—we seem instead to allow the pendulum to swing back and forth between the two different views.

Table 2
**Comparison of Paper-based Claim-processing System
with an Electronic System**

Issue	Current Paper-based System	Electronic System
Consumer fills out claim forms	Yes, for each visit to a medical provider, each piece of medical equipment, and each medical procedure or test	No, claims can be filed electronically by the provider
Consumer photocopies all medical bills	Yes, for each visit to a medical provider, each piece of medical equipment, and each medical procedure or test	No, bills can be permanently maintained on a computer or an electronic card
Cost	Enormously expensive in terms of the cost of paper-based claim-filing, record keeping, and personnel	Potential savings of billions of dollars
Consumer mails claim forms (in some cases, to both primary and secondary insurers)	Yes, for each visit to a medical provider, each piece of medical equipment, and each medical test or procedure	No, all claims filed electronically

Table 2 (Continued)

Issue	Current Paper-based System	Electronic System
Consumer collects documentation, if necessary, for all routine claim problems	Yes, whenever the insurer denies a claim pending receipt of additional documentation or information	No, requests for additional documentation for routine claim problems directed to the provider
Consumer files claim appeals in regard to routine claim problems	Yes, whenever the insurer denies a claim pending receipt of additional documentation or information	No, claim appeals are filed electronically by the medical provider, not by the consumer
Consumer maintains extensive records and copies of bills, claims, and documents	Yes, for each visit to a medical provider, each piece of medical equipment, and each medical procedure or test	No, records permanently maintained on a computer or on an electronic card
Speed	Claim-processing may require four weeks for a routine claim; if a secondary insurer is involved, the process may require a month or two	Claims filed by the provider and received by the insurer within a few seconds; payment made electronically

At times over the past few years, Americans have seemed convinced that only government intervention could provide a solution to health insurance problems. State and federal legislatures then began to pass laws—and government agencies began to issue regulations—to control the health insurance system. However, because of the existing philosophical debate, government efforts at regulation have often been criticized, and are generally limited.

For example, while there have been recent efforts in several states to guarantee the availability of individual health insurance policies to all citizens, regardless of existing illnesses or disabilities, the process was never completed. Equal access to health insurance was sometimes guaranteed, but at the same time the government allowed the free market system to determine premiums. The result is that while health insurance policies may officially be available to all individuals in some states, the premiums for such policies may be so high that they are out of the reach of many consumers.

At other times, the pendulum seems to swing in the opposite direction, away from government intervention. The government then begins to eliminate some of the existing laws and regulations in order to allow health insurers to operate in a free market setting. However, because of the continuing philosophical debate, some of the laws and regulations are left in place, making it difficult for the free market system to operate efficiently. Soon, if costs escalate and many consumers are left without health insurance coverage, there's a demand once again for new laws and new government regulations.

Thus, the cycle continues. There's a constant shift from one approach to the other, without giving either government regulation or the free market system a real opportunity to demonstrate its effectiveness. As a result, the health insurance maze becomes more complex as the years pass.

Recent proposals to reform the American health insurance system have focused a great deal of attention on health insurance issues. However, given the current philosophical debate, and the lack of effective solutions to existing problems, I don't think that consumers can depend either on the government or on the free market to solve the problems inherent in the health insurance system at this point. Thus, it's important that consumers develop the tools they need to deal effectively with health insurance problems on their own.

2

Understanding the Language of Health Insurance

All fields have a technical language of their own. In order to follow a conversation between attorneys, biologists, chemists, engineers, or automobile mechanics, you need to be able to understand the technical terminology used in those fields. That's true of the health insurance field, as well. In fact, the health insurance field has developed a highly specialized, technical language all its own. In order to deal with health insurance problems effectively, you'll need to understand that language.

These days, communication among consumers and doctors, hospitals, laboratories, health insurance companies, and government agencies is often conducted by mail, with few opportunities to ask for explanations. That makes the need to understand the technical language of health insurance even more important. In this chapter we'll review a number of technical terms and phrases that are frequently used in communications between insurers and consumers.

TECHNICAL TERMS USED IN CLAIM PROCESSING

Several years ago, I dealt with a problem in which an insurance company had denied a series of claims for the treatment of depression. The claims covered a number of sessions with a psychiatrist. The bills amounted to more than a thousand dollars, and additional sessions had already been scheduled.

When I reviewed the statements from the insurer explaining why the claims had been denied, I noticed that the company had requested a copy of an accident report. Since that seemed to be a particularly odd request, given the nature of the treatment, I called a supervisor at the insurance company. As I reviewed the case with the supervisor, I discovered that the consumer had written the word **"therapy"** on the claim form under "Type of Illness or Treatment."

Some insurance companies—including the company involved in processing this particular claim—use the term "therapy" to refer only to **physical therapy.** Therapy sessions with a psychologist or psychiatrist to treat mental or emotional illnesses are generally referred to technically as **"outpatient treatment for mental illness."** When the claims processor saw the word "therapy" on the claim form, she had apparently assumed that the claim involved physical therapy. She then requested an accident report, on the assumption that the need for physical therapy was the result of an accident.

In the meantime, the claims were temporarily denied, pending the receipt of either an accident report or a letter of explanation confirming that the physical therapy was not related to an accident. When the claims were re-filed with the phrase "outpatient treatment for mental illness" instead of "therapy" written under "Type of Illness or Treatment" on the claim form, they were paid without difficulty.

Many health insurance claim problems turn out to be the result of similar misunderstandings related to the use of technical terms and phrases. In order to communicate effectively with an insurer, or to understand the letters or statements that insurers send to consumers, it's often necessary to understand that terminology.

The first thing consumers may notice when they look at a letter from an insurance company is that doctors, laboratories, testing centers, and hospitals are now generally referred to in the health insurance field as **providers, medical providers,** or **providers of service.** If the providers are part of an insurance company's network—doctors, laboratories, hospitals, and testing centers that have agreed to follow specific insurance company rules—they are generally referred to as **network providers** or **plan providers.**

In addition, insurance companies now generally request **documentation** rather than statements of explanation to support a claim. Documentation might include a letter from a doctor explaining the **medical necessity**—the medical need or purpose—of a particular treatment or procedure (sometimes referred to as a **Letter of Medical Necessity**) or an **operative report** (a detailed description of the procedures followed during an operation, usually written by the physician who performed the surgery). Documentation might also include a detailed or itemized bill from a hospital, doctor, testing center, or laboratory.

Furthermore, insurance companies no longer send letters of explanation to consumers to explain their determination of the amount of reimbursement provided in relation to a claim. Instead, they send an **EOBS (Explanation of Benefits Statement)** after a claim has been processed.

There is no universal Explanation of Benefits Statement form, and the placement of particular information may vary from insurer to insurer. However, all Explanation of Benefits Statements generally contain the name of the policyholder—the person who is insured—the patient's name if the patient is different than the policyholder, the policyholder's identification number, the name of the provider, the date of service or treatment, the amount of the bill, and the amount of reimbursement provided by the insurer. An Explanation of Benefits Statement may also include an explanation of the way reimbursement was determined. In addition, there may be specific notes on any charges that were excluded (See Table 3).

Table 3 represents an Explanation of Benefits Statement in a situation involving an office visit to a doctor. The entire $100 charge was considered eligible for payment. Since the deductible had been previously satisfied in the case illustrated in Table 3, and since the policy provided for payment at the 80% rate, $80 of the bill was paid by the insurer.

Table 3
Sample Explanation of Benefits Statement

Insured: (Name of the policyholder)
Patient: (Name of patient if different from policyholder)
ID Number: (Policyholder's identification number)
Date Processed: (Date the claim was processed)

Medical Provider	Date of Service	Type of Service	Amount of Bill
(Provider's Name)	(Date)	Office Visit	$100
Eligible	**Not Eligible**	**Percentage**	**Deductible**
$100	0	80%	0
Amount Paid	**Sent To**	**Balance**	**Notes**
$ 80	Consumer	$20	

In this case, the check was sent to the consumer, who had presumably already paid the medical bill in full. The $20 balance refers to the **co-payment,** the amount that the consumer is expected to pay out-of-pocket, without reimbursement.

If treatment was provided by a **network provider** or a **plan provider,** the Explanation of Benefits Statement might also include a note about the amount of the original bill that was determined to be ineligible. Table 4 represents an Explanation of Benefits Statement in a situation that involved an office visit to a doctor where the doctor was part of the insurance company's network (See Table 4).

Although the original bill illustrated in Table 4 was $100— the doctor's standard charge—only $80 was considered eligible for payment according to network rules. The deductible had been previously satisfied.

Table 4
Sample Explanation of Benefits Statement Where the Provider Is Part of a Plan Network

Insured: (Name of the policyholder)
Patient: (Name of patient if different from policyholder)
ID Number: (Policyholder's identification number)
Date Processed: (Date the claim was processed)

Medical Provider	Date of Service	Type of Service	Amount of Bill
(Provider's Name)	(Date)	Office Visit	$100
Eligible	**Not Eligible**	**Percentage**	**Deductible**
$80	$20	80%	0
Amount Paid	**Sent To**	**Balance**	**Notes**
$64	Provider	$16	Network Provider

In the case illustrated by Table 4, the policy provided for payment of 80% of the eligible amount. Thus, $64 of the bill was paid by the insurer. The check was sent to the provider, since the provider is part of the insurance company's network.

The $16 balance noted in Table 4 refers to the co-payment, the amount that the consumer is expected to pay out-of-pocket. Since the provider is a part of the plan network, and agreed to follow network rules, the payment in this case represents 80% of the $80 eligible amount. The consumer is not generally responsible for the amount—$20 in this case—that was considered ineligible.

An EOBS may also contain computer-generated technical

terms or phrases in the comments section, usually found in the middle or at the bottom of the form. Some of those terms may be particularly confusing at times. The phrase **not medically necessary**—sometimes printed on an EOBS as an explanation for a claim denial—is a good illustration of the problem.

Many insurance companies use the phrase "not medically necessary" in two very different ways. In some cases, the phrase may be used to mean that the company is unable to determine whether or not a treatment is medically necessary under policy rules—and thus eligible for reimbursement under the policy—and that additional documentation is required before the determination can be made. In other cases, the phrase may be used to mean that a decision has been made that the treatment or service is not considered medically necessary under the terms of the policy and is thus not covered. Unfortunately, it's sometimes very difficult for consumers to determine how the phrase is being used in a particular EOBS.

For example, several years ago I helped a reader of my newspaper column solve a problem in which a claim for extensive surgery had apparently been denied. According to the insurance company's EOBS the surgery was considered "not medically necessary." Since the bills amounted to more than $20,000, the reader was obviously deeply concerned. I spoke with the surgeon, and he felt strongly that the surgery was not only necessary from a medical point of view, it was essential.

When I discussed the situation with a supervisor at the insurance company, I discovered that the company was using the term "not medically necessary" in this case to mean that additional documentation was needed before making a determination on the claim. The company's procedures required that an operative report and a more detailed hospital bill be filed in cases involving major surgery before the company could refer the claim to a medical consultant to make a decision on the issue of medical necessity. In that sense, the phrase "not medically necessary" referred to an administrative or procedural issue rather than to the medical need for the surgery.

The insurance company had a limited number of computerized codes that personnel could choose from when processing a claim. The company had a code that printed the words "not medically necessary" on an EOBS, but there was no computer code to print a statement such as, "We need an operative report and a detailed hospital bill before we can process this claim further." There apparently wasn't even a computer code to print the words "Insufficient documentation."

According to the insurance company supervisor, the company's records indicated that several letters had been sent requesting the required documentation, but that there had been no response. Thus, the claim had been placed temporarily on hold. However, when I discussed the issue with the doctor and with hospital representatives, they were certain that they had never received any requests for additional information or documentation.

Once the problem was clear, it was a simple matter to ask the doctor and the hospital to fax the appropriate documentation directly to the insurance company supervisor and to ask the supervisor to have the claim reviewed as quickly as possible. Once that process was completed, the claim was approved for payment within 48 hours.

After the problem had been solved, I had an opportunity to discuss the case with an executive at the insurance company. He was not aware that the company was printing a "not medically necessary" statement on the EOBS when the documentation was incomplete, and he agreed to make certain that additional computer codes were added to allow other, more appropriate, messages to be printed in the future.

This case is a good illustration of the difficulties involved in understanding the meaning of the technical terms and phrases sometimes used by insurers to communicate with consumers, and of the need for consumers to understand the meaning of as many technical terms and phrases as possible. Although this particular problem was easily solved, it's not always possible to find a solution to a major health insurance problem so quickly, or to persuade an insurance company of the need to change its claim-processing procedures. Fortunately, the cooperation of the doctor, the hospital representatives, and the insurance company supervisors and executives involved in the case made that kind of solution possible.

In addition to the confusion that results from the use of technical terminology, at times some insurance companies also seem to have difficulty communicating basic information to consumers. For example, I helped a reader solve a problem several years ago that involved a claim for ambulance service. The patient was covered by Medicare and by a secondary insurance policy. Medicare had paid a large portion of the cost of the ambulance service, but the secondary insurer had declined to pay the difference—approximately $150—between the Medicare payment and the original bill. The secondary insurer's explanation for declining to provide payment was that "maximum benefits" had already been provided for "hospital charges" under the "hospital service plan." In addition, the letter of explanation from the insurer claimed that the policy did not provide coverage for ambulance service.

I found the insurer's explanations so confusing that I had to call an executive at the insurance company to review the technical terms that the company was using. As it turned out, although the letter of explanation from the insurer stated that the policy did not cover ambulance service, the policy did in fact provide coverage for such services. In addition, the phrase "maximum benefits" referred to the Medicare payment, not to a payment by the secondary insurer, "hospital charges" referred to ambulance service, and "hospital service plan" referred to Medicare.

As I eventually discovered, what the insurer meant to communicate was that the policy provided for payment for ambulance service only up to a specific amount. Since the Medicare payment had already exceeded that amount, the secondary insurer was not obligated under the policy to make any additional payments. Apparently, if Medicare had not made a payment, the secondary insurer would have done so, up to the limit provided by the policy.

I recently helped another reader deal with a situation that also illustrates the difficulties that insurance companies sometimes have in communicating basic information to consumers. In this case, the reader was covered by a private insurer. He had been in the hospital, and had been treated for a serious condition by several different medical specialists on the same day. The insurer, however, only paid one of the bills. The insurer's explanation was that the policy provided coverage for only "one provider per day."

When I checked with the insurer, I discovered that the problem was really quite different. One of the claims had apparently been submitted without a diagnosis. According to an executive at the insurance company, the diagnosis that was eventually submitted was the same as the diagnosis on a claim for the same date that had already been paid. Since the diagnoses were identical, the second claim was denied. However, after review, the insurer determined that the reader was being treated for "multiple conditions" and that reimbursement for treatments by several specialists on the same day was thus appropriate. Interestingly, although the insurer's original explanation was that the policy provided coverage for only one provider per day, the policy did not contain any such provision. However, the comment that the policy paid for only "one provider per day" was one of the computer-generated statements available to be printed on an EOBS to explain the denial of a claim.

I think there's a desperate need to improve communication between insurers and consumers, particularly in terms of the messages in letters from insurers to consumers and on Explanation of Benefits Statements. Part of the difficulty is that those messages often make use of technical terminology. In addition, the messages in letters and on EOBS are often limited, are usually computer-generated, and are not written on a personal basis. Table 5 helps illustrate some of the technical terms that are frequently used by insurers in letters to consumers and in EOBS (See Table 5).

Table 5
Technical Terms Used in Claim-processing

Technical Term	Meaning
EOBS (Explanation of Benefits Statement)	A statement sent from the insurance company to the patient; lists charges, dates of service, and reimbursement
Medical Provider (Provider, Provider of Service)	A doctor, testing center, or hospital that provides treatment or medical services
Network or Plan Provider	A doctor, testing center, or hospital that is part of the insurance company's network and that has agreed to follow network rules
Therapy	A term that often refers to physical therapy, not to psychological or psychiatric treatment
Outpatient Treatment for Mental Illness	Therapy offered by a mental health provider such as a psychologist or psychiatrist on an outpatient basis
Documentation	The paperwork that insurers require before processing a claim; may include a letter of medical necessity, an operative report, or an itemized bill
Operative Report	A detailed report of the procedures performed during surgery

Table 5 (Continued)

Technical Term	Meaning
Letter of Medical Necessity	A letter from a doctor explaining why a specific medical test, treatment, or type of medical equipment is necessary
Not Medically Necessary	A phrase used to mean either that a claim cannot be processed until all of the required documentation has been provided, or that the insurer has determined that the claim does not meet the policy requirements, and is thus not considered a covered expense under the terms of the policy

TECHNICAL TERMS USED TO DESCRIBE HEALTH INSURANCE PLANS

In addition to the technical terms that are used in claim-processing, there are a number of technical terms that are used to describe the current types of health insurance plans. The health insurance plan with which you're probably most familiar is the **traditional plan,** sometimes called a **fee-for-service plan** or an **indemnity plan.** In a traditional plan, you can choose any medical provider—doctor, hospital, testing center, or laboratory—you wish. Following treatment, you pay the bill and then send it to your insurer for reimbursement. Traditional plans are available in the form of both **individual** and **group plans.**

The terms "individual" and "group" in this sense do not refer to the question of whether a particular insurance plan provides coverage for an individual or a family. Rather, the terms refer to the question of whether the person is covered through an insurance policy that has been purchased as an individual, or through an insurance plan as part of a larger group such as a corporation, a business, or an association. Thus, either an individual or a group policy may provide coverage for a single person or for an entire family.

There are also different types of **managed care** plans, sometimes referred to as **MCOs (Managed Care Organizations)**. Although managed care plans may differ significantly in terms of policy rules, such plans have certain characteristics in common. For example, managed care plans generally provide maximum benefits only when you choose doctors, hospitals, testing centers, or laboratories from a list of **network providers** (sometimes referred to as **participating providers** or **plan providers**). In some cases, the doctors, the testing center, and the laboratory may be located in a single building. In other cases, they may be located in different buildings or in different areas, connected through their participation in the managed care plan's network.

In addition to offering coverage for the standard types of medical expenses, managed care plans usually also offer coverage for a variety of preventive services. Those services may include an annual physical exam, vaccinations, and routine screening tests. However, access to specialists and to expensive medical tests in a managed care plan is generally available only with the approval of the **primary care physician,** the doctor who is responsible for coordinating all of the medical care for an individual.

HMOs (Health Maintenance Organizations) and **PPOs (Preferred Provider Organizations)** are among the most common types of managed care plans. Health Maintenance Organizations generally expect participants to use network providers, except in special situations. Some HMOs have **POS (Point-of-Service) Options.** Although the details differ from plan to plan, a POS Option generally allows participants to consult out-of-network providers in some cases and still qualify for partial reimbursement.

PPOs have a provider network, as well, and also permit participants to occasionally use providers who are not part of the network and still receive partial reimbursement. In that sense, a PPO and an HMO with a Point-of-Service Option are similar in some respects. However, there are differences, as well (See Chapter 7 for a more complete discussion of this issue).

There are also **self-funded plans,** offered by plan sponsors. A self-funded plan might be sponsored by a corporation for its employees, by a union or association for its members, or by a state or municipal government agency. Although there may be an insurance company involved in a self-funded plan, the company generally acts as the **plan administrator** rather than as the insurer. In that case, the insurance company does not determine the plan rules. Rather, the insurance company makes benefit-related decisions on the basis of the rules set by the plan sponsor.

Self-funded plans vary considerably, both in terms of benefits and structure. For example, some self-funded plans are set up as traditional plans, while others are set up as managed care plans. However, unlike traditional plans or managed care plans established by insurance companies, self-funded plans are generally regulated under **ERISA**—the federal **Employee Retirement Income Security Act**—in terms of benefit-related issues, rather than under state law. (See Chapter 6 for a more detailed discussion of self-funded plans.)

There are also a number of government-sponsored health insurance programs, including **Medicare** and **Medicaid.** Medicare is sponsored by the federal government and provides health insurance coverage for senior citizens and for some children and adults with disabilities. It is regulated by HCFA, the Health Care Financing Administration. Medicaid is sponsored jointly by the federal and state governments and provides coverage for people whose income is below the poverty line and for many children with disabilities (See Table 6).

Table 6
Technical Terms Used to Describe Health Insurance Plans

Type of Insurance Plan	Description
Traditional Plan (Indemnity Plan, Fee-for-Service Plan)	A plan in which the consumer chooses the doctor, laboratory, testing center, or hospital, pays the bill, and sends the claim to the insurer for reimbursement
Managed Care Plan	A plan such as an HMO or PPO in which participants must generally use medical providers that are part of the plan network in order to obtain maximum benefits
HMO with POS Option	A managed care plan that allows participants to occasionally consult out-of-network providers and still obtain partial reimbursement
Self-funded Plan	A plan established by a corporation, by a union or association for its members, or by a state or municipal government agency; if an insurer is involved, the insurer acts as plan administrator

TECHNICAL TERMS USED TO DESCRIBE PLAN BENEFITS

Historically, health insurance plans had their origin in coverage for hospital-based treatment. Over the years, additional benefits were added from time to time. At first, those added benefits could be purchased separately as **riders** to the original plan. As the years went by, in many cases some of those riders were routinely added to the standard plan until eventually both the original plan and the riders began to be offered as a single group. However, rather than being fully integrated into the plan, the added provisions were sometimes incorporated as separate benefit provisions, such as "major medical" or "basic benefits." That group of benefit provisions, combined with the original hospitalization policy, appears to have evolved into the type of individual and group health insurance plans often provided by insurance companies today.

As a result, although consumers who purchase a health insurance policy at this point may be under the impression that they are purchasing a fully integrated policy—with a single deductible and a single set of rules—the reality is that they may be purchasing a group of separate benefit provisions offered as a single policy. Each of those provisions is designed to provide coverage for a different kind of medical treatment, procedure, or type of equipment, and each policy provision may have a different deductible and may follow different rules. For example, many health insurance policies currently include separate provisions for **hospitalization, surgery, basic benefits, major medical, durable medical equipment,** and for the treatment of **mental and emotional illnesses.** Policies may also include a variety of separate riders, providing coverage for eyeglasses, prescription medications, and other benefits.

The hospitalization provision and the surgical provision—sometimes referred to as **hospital-surgical**—generally represents the original type of policy offered by insurers decades earlier. It provides coverage for inpatient hospital treatment, including the cost of hospital facilities, nursing care, room, and food. **Basic benefits** may include coverage for specific medical tests, ambulance service, and oxygen. Basic benefits may be paid even when the **yearly deductible**—the amount you must pay each year before the insurance company will begin to reimburse you for claims—has not yet been met.

For example, let's assume that you go to the doctor because you've injured your ankle, and the doctor takes an X-ray. If your policy has a deductible, as most policies do, and if this is your first visit to a doctor for the calendar year, the policy may not provide reimbursement for the doctor's visit since the yearly deductible has not yet been met. However, the policy may nevertheless provide reimbursement for the X-ray under the basic benefits provision.

Major medical benefits refer to coverage for treatment by a doctor and for medical tests that are not covered under the basic benefits portion of the policy. Treatment in a hospital emergency room, same-day surgery at a hospital center, or medical tests conducted in a hospital setting on an outpatient basis are often included under the major medical provision, as well. Such hospital-based treatments and tests are not generally considered part of inpatient care—even though they may take place within a hospital—because the patient is not scheduled to stay overnight.

Depending on the policy, major medical claims may be reimbursed by the insurer at the 50%, 60%, 70%, or 80% rate, with the 50%, 40%, 30%, or 20% balance paid by the individual. Such policies are sometimes described as 50/50, 60/40, 70/30, or 80/20 plans. The first number refers to the percentage of the bill for which the insurance policy will generally provide reimbursement; the second number refers to the percentage of the bill that is generally paid for by the consumer. For example, if a doctor's bill is $100 and the insurance policy provides for payment of major medical claims at the 80% rate (an 80/20 plan), the insurer will generally provide reimbursement of $80. You will be expected to pay the $20 balance (the co-payment or co-insurance amount).

Major medical benefits don't generally begin until you have met the yearly deductible. However, that deductible is usually separate from the deductible established for hospital or surgical benefits. Thus, although you may have been in the hospital earlier in the year, you may still need to meet the yearly major medical deductible separately. In the same way, although you may have already met the major medical deductible for the year, you may still need to meet a separate hospital-surgical deductible—if your policy includes such a deductible—if you are hospitalized.

Insurance policies that include **family coverage**—coverage for dependents—also often include a provision for a **family deductible** under the major medical portion of the policy. Although the details differ from policy to policy, the general concept of the family deductible is that once several individuals in a family have each met the individual deductible, all other family members are assumed to have met that deductible as well. At that point, the other family members receive coverage under the major medical provision beginning with their first medical bill of the year. However, even when the yearly deductible or the family deductible has been met in regard to major medical claims, you will still have to pay the co-payment or co-insurance.

Many insurance policies also include a provision for a **yearly co-payment maximum.** That limits co-payments for the year. Under the yearly co-payment maximum, once you have paid the co-payment for a predetermined level of medical bills—between $2,000 and $5,000 in major medical bills during the year in many cases, depending on the policy—all additional major medical claims are generally paid at the 100% rate.

However, payment at the 100% rate doesn't necessarily mean that the entire medical bill will be paid. Rather, it means that once you have met the yearly major medical co-payment maximum, the insurer will pay 100% of the **UCR**—the **Usual and Customary Rate**—for expenses covered by the policy. The UCR is generally determined by a statistical analysis of providers' charges for a particular procedure, in a specific geographic area.

That analysis is usually based on data collected by insurance companies in relation to charges for each type of medical test, service, or treatment. The data is entered into a computer database and is generally subdivided by state, geographic region, or ZIP code. Once the process has been completed and an array of charges has been established for a particular procedure, reimbursement in relation to claims is usually limited to the UCR, regardless of the actual amount of the medical provider's bill.

The determination of the UCR is directly affected by the **percentile system.** Although a health insurance policy may provide for reimbursement of major medical claims at the 80% rate (an 80/20 plan), the amount that will be paid by the insurer may depend on the specific percentile provided for in the policy. (See Chapter 4 for a more complete discussion of the UCR and percentile systems.)

In some policies, the amount of reimbursement may also be limited by both the **yearly benefit maximum** (the maximum amount of reimbursement available under major medical during a single calendar year) and the **lifetime benefit maximum** (the maximum amount of reimbursement available under the policy during a person's lifetime). Those amounts, of course, vary from policy to policy.

In addition, some insurance policies may have a separate provision for durable medical equipment. That provision relates to coverage for such equipment as manual and power wheelchairs, crutches, and walkers. Traditionally, only certain types of medical equipment have been covered by health insurance policies. Other types of equipment are generally excluded from coverage. For example, many health insurance policies provide coverage for both manual and power wheelchairs under provisions for durable medical equipment. However, other types of related equipment—wheelchair ramps, wheelchair lifts, reduced effort steering for a car or van, a specially adapted computer, an accessible shower—are rarely covered by health insurance policies, even though they may be directly related to a medical condition.

Preventive care—treatment for the prevention of illnesses—is not usually covered by traditional health insurance policies. Such policies are generally designed to pay only for the treatment of existing illnesses or conditions, rather than for their prevention. However, managed care plans often include coverage for such preventive services as routine yearly physical exams, vaccinations, and routine screening tests.

Benefits for the treatment of mental and emotional illness may be covered by a separate provision in some health insurance policies. That provision generally includes coverage for the treatment of depression, anxiety, Schizophrenia, bipolar disorder, and similar illnesses or conditions. Treatments in relation to drug and alcohol problems may also be included in that category under some insurance policies. (See Table 7 for a list of technical terms used to describe plan benefits and for the definition of each of those terms.)

There may be different rules for coverage for the treatment of mental and emotional illness, both in terms of treatment in a therapist's office (outpatient treatment for mental illness) and hospital-based treatment (inpatient treatment for mental illness). For example, some health insurance policies have traditionally had different yearly or lifetime benefit maximums in terms of coverage for the treatment of mental illness as compared to coverage for the treatment of physical illness. However, the recently enacted federal Mental Health Parity Act requires changes in the rules related to yearly and lifetime benefit maximums for physical and mental illnesses. (See Chapter 4 for a discussion of issues related to mental health parity).

Table 7
Technical Terms Used to Describe Plan Benefits

Technical Term	Meaning
Co-Payment or Co-Insurance	The percentage of each medical bill that you must pay, once the deductible has been met
Yearly Individual Deductible	The amount that you need to pay each year before the insurer will generally begin to pay major medical claims

Table 7 (Continued)

Technical Term	Meaning
Preventive Care	Vaccinations, routine physical exams, and screening tests
Durable Medical Equipment	Equipment such as a power wheelchair or crutches
Family Coverage	Coverage for dependents
Family Deductible	Once several family members have met the yearly deductible, the deductible is assumed to have been met by all other family members
Yearly Co-Payment Maximum	The maximum amount you need to pay for covered major medical claims each year; once that amount has been reached, no co-payments are generally required, and claims for covered expenses are paid at the 100% rate
Yearly Benefit Maximum	That maximum amount of reimbursement that a policy will provide in terms of benefits during a calendar year
Lifetime Benefit Maximum	The maximum amount of reimbursement that a policy will provide in terms of benefits during a person's lifetime

Table 7 (Continued)

Technical Term	Meaning
Basic Benefits	Benefits for some X-rays and tests; in some cases, reimbursement may be provided even when the yearly deductible has not been met
Major Medical Benefits	Benefits for doctors' bills and for tests that are not covered under basic benefits
Usual and Customary Rate (the UCR)	The maximum amount of reimbursement an insurer will generally consider for a particular treatment or test
Percentile	The level of the array of charges at which reimbursement will be considered
Hospital Benefits (Inpatient), Hospital-Surgical Benefits	Benefits for an overnight stay in a hospital; includes coverage for nursing care, room, and food
Hospital Benefits (Outpatient)	Benefits for treatment in a hospital emergency room or a hospital same-day surgery facility, or for tests performed in a hospital on an outpatient basis; claims may be covered under major medical

SUMMARY

At this point, we've reviewed many of the technical terms and phrases that are commonly used in interactions between consumers and health insurers. An understanding of those terms represents one of the most important tools for dealing successfully with your health insurance.

However, it's important to remember that some health insurance companies may have their own definitions for some of these terms, or may use specific terms in a somewhat different way. If that occurs, just ask an insurance company representative for the meaning of the particular technical term as it's being used by the company.

Now that you understand many of the technical terms and phrases used in the health insurance field, we can begin to focus on the details of preventing and dealing with specific claim problems. If you forget the exact meaning of a technical term or phrase at any point, you'll find it listed in the glossary.

3

Developing a Systematic Approach to Dealing with Health Insurance Claims

Benjamin Franklin once wrote that "nothing can be said to be certain, except death and taxes." If he were alive today, Franklin might have added health insurance problems to that list. In fact, health insurance problems are one of the most common types of consumer problems that Americans face these days. The way consumers deal with those problems can either intensify them, or can set the stage for a solution.

For example, I'm sure you've heard of people who keep their medical bills in an old shoe box and file the claims whenever they get around to it. The difficulty with that kind of approach is that when the person finally does get around to sorting through the bills, so much time has passed and so many bills have accumulated that a great deal of work is usually required to figure out how to file each claim. Knowing that the work is likely to be enormously time-consuming may lead to a decision to put it off even longer.

However, many insurance policies require that claims be filed within one year of the date of treatment. When the person finally begins to review the medical bills, the time limit may already have expired for some of the bills, and other bills may no longer make sense. Either the person is unable to remember if the bills represent photocopies—where the original bills were previously filed—or is unable to find the matching bills and EOBS from the primary insurer, making it impossible to file the claims with a secondary insurer. The result is that the claims are not filed properly—or not filed at all—and the person loses money.

In contrast, while developing a systematic approach to dealing with claims may not be particularly exciting, it can make claim-filing easier and more efficient and can save both time and money. It can also help you prevent claim problems from occurring, and it can make it easier for you to deal with the problems that do occur.

You might want to think of dealing with health insurance claims as a part-time job. In fact, given the high cost of medical care these days, and the importance of obtaining the benefits to which you are entitled from your insurance policy, you may find that it's a part-time job that's quite worthwhile from an economic point of view.

THE SIX STEP APPROACH TO DEALING WITH HEALTH INSURANCE CLAIMS

Developing a systematic approach to dealing with health insurance claims involves six steps

1. setting up an information file;
2. using the predetermination of benefits process;
3. establishing an efficient claim-filing system;
4. setting up a record keeping system;
5. developing a method for filing claim appeals with insurers;
6. establishing a system for requesting help from government agencies or private organizations.

STEP ONE: SETTING UP AN INFORMATION FILE

Setting up an information file involves writing down questions about your current health insurance policy and then recording the answers to those questions. There are a number of questions and answers that should be included in any information file (See Table 8).

Table 8
Sample Information File

Question	Answer
What is the name, mailing address, and phone number of your insurer?	
What is your insurance company identification number?	
How much is the individual yearly deductible (and the family deductible, if you have family coverage)?	
What are the yearly and lifetime benefit maximums?	
What kinds of preventive care (routine physical exams, vaccinations, screening tests) are covered?	
What special rules exist for reimbursement for the treatment of mental and emotional illnesses?	
What services or treatments require pre-authorization?	
What are the steps for obtaining pre-authorization?	
If there is a network of medical providers, where can the up-to-date list of those providers be found?	

Table 8 (Continued)

Question	Answer
Does your policy offer reimbursement for services performed by non-network providers?	
What is the procedure for obtaining reimbursement for bills from non-network providers?	
How much is the co-payment or co-insurance amount (the amount of each bill that you have to pay once the yearly deductible is met)?	
How much is the yearly co-payment maximum (the total amount your medical bills need to reach before the insurer will pay bills for covered expenses at the 100% rate)?	
What percentile is used in the determination of the UCR in terms of major medical claims?	
What secondary insurance benefits are offered under the policy, and to whom in the family do those benefits apply?	

Table 8 (Continued)

Question	Answer
What are the rules that relate to using the predetermination of benefits process? (See Step Two)	
If you have children, and you have more than one insurance policy with family coverage, which policy is primary for the children?	
What are the steps involved in appealing a claim that has been denied?	

Of course, you'll also want to add your own questions and answers to your information file. In addition, if you talk with a particularly helpful supervisor or executive at your insurance company at some point, list that person's name and telephone number in your information file, as well. If you have both a primary and a secondary insurer, create a separate information file for each one.

Many people wait until they need this kind of information before they try to obtain answers to their questions. Unfortunately, that approach does not often work very well, and may lead to difficulty if you're unable to obtain the information you need when you have to make a decision. Listing the information in advance in an information file guarantees that it will be available whenever it's needed. Since the booklets provided by insurance companies are not always clear, listing the answers to questions in advance also offers an opportunity to call or write to the insurer to request additional information in terms of specific benefits.

STEP TWO: PREDETERMINATION OF BENEFITS

The predetermination of benefits process allows the medical provider—at the consumer's request—to send the insurance company a statement listing a proposed treatment or test, or the proposed purchase of medical equipment. Within a few weeks, the insurance company will generally respond with a statement of the amount of reimbursement the company will usually provide for that test, procedure, or equipment.

That process offers the consumer valuable information. It makes it possible for the consumer to review the cost and possible reimbursement for treatments or tests in advance, and allows the consumer to make an appropriate decision before the test or procedure is performed. In addition, if there's a significant difference between the estimated cost and possible reimbursement—or if the insurer determines that the test or procedure is not covered under the policy—the predetermination of benefits process offers an opportunity for the consumer to discuss the economic issues with the doctor or the insurer in advance.

The predetermination of benefits process may be helpful in all non-emergency situations that involve significant cost, such as elective surgery, expensive medical tests, or the purchase of medical equipment. In such cases, the predetermination of benefits process can help to prevent situations in which the consumer may be caught in the middle between the medical provider and the insurer.

For example, several years ago I reviewed a claim with a reader of my newspaper column involving a situation in which an individual had several small growths surgically removed at the same time. When the surgery was completed, the surgeon sent the patient a bill that reflected the removal of each of the growths.

However, since the surgeries were performed at the same time, the insurer provided reimbursement for less than half of the total bill in terms of the removal of the second growth on the grounds that the removal of that growth was incidental to the removal of the first growth. That left the individual with a large bill for which he was responsible. The predetermination of benefits process would have given the consumer information about billing and reimbursement in advance. That would have made it possible for the consumer to discuss those issues with the provider and the insurer prior to surgery.

Such cases, in which the consumer is caught between a medical provider and an insurer, are unfortunately not unusual. There seem to be a number of situations in which no clearly agreed upon standards exist for how bills should be structured or how reimbursement should be provided. At present, medical providers make their own decisions on billing, and insurers make their own decisions on reimbursement. Since consumers are generally considered to be responsible for the entire medical bill—regardless of the amount of reimbursement provided by an insurer—such situations can result in significant economic difficulty for consumers. That's why it's so important to make use of the predetermination of benefits process whenever possible.

Of course, since the predetermination of benefits process can take several weeks, it's not useful to ask a doctor to file such a request in an emergency situation or in a situation in which you need the answers to a specific medical test as quickly as possible. In addition, there's generally no value to the process if you're a participant in a managed care program and the provider is part of the managed care plan network (See Chapter 7).

However, in other cases where the test or procedure is elective or where you are willing to consider alternatives—for example, repairing an existing piece of medical equipment rather than purchasing new equipment—the process can be extremely helpful from an economic point of view. You need to be aware, though, that although many insurers will offer a detailed response to a predetermination of benefits request, some insurers may offer only a general statement, and will make an official determination only when the claim itself is filed. Check with your insurer to determine their specific policy rules for the predetermination of benefits process.

STEP THREE: ESTABLISHING AN EFFICIENT CLAIM-FILING SYSTEM

Setting up an efficient claim-filing system may save you a great deal of time and effort in the long run. For example, many people fill out a new claim form by hand each time they file a health insurance claim. That's time-consuming and is often unnecessary. My experience is that many insurers will accept claim forms that are computer-generated or photocopied as long as the signature on the form is original.

If your insurer accepts photocopies of their claim forms, you need to fill out the basic information—name, address, and so on—only once. After that, you can photocopy the completed form, and you can run off as many copies as you wish. That way, all you have to do is sign the form and send it in with your claims. If you have a computer and your insurer accepts computer-generated forms, you can make use of programs that will print a health insurance claim form directly from the computer using a database that automatically fills in the basic information.

If you have both a primary and a secondary insurer, you may be able to save additional time by using a universal claim form. That may allow you to file claims with a single form, instead of filling out different types of forms for each insurer. Although private insurance companies are not required to accept universal claim forms, many private insurance companies do so at this point. Universal claim forms can generally be obtained from a business products supply company.

Whichever method you use to fill out your claim forms, it's essential to make certain that all of the information is accurate and is written or typed clearly. Since rules vary, it's important to check with your insurance company to determine its policy on accepting computer-generated, photocopied, or universal claim forms before purchasing a computer program or universal claim forms, or before photocopying insurance company claim forms.

Another way to make claim-filing easier is to fill out only part of the claim form. In addition to asking for basic information—

your name, address, insurance identification number—health insurance claim forms also generally include a section that requests information about the medical provider, the date of treatment, the nature of the illness, the diagnosis, and the amount of the bill. However, you may not need to fill out that section of the claim form if you are attaching the medical bill, since the bill itself generally contains all the required information.

If your insurer accepts medical bills in place of fully completed claim forms—as many insurers will—you need to fill out only the basic information on the form. Write "See Attached Bill" in the section of the form that requests information about the doctor, the date of treatment, and the diagnosis, and attach a copy of the medical bill to the claim form.

It's essential to photocopy that medical bill for your records before mailing in the claim and to keep those photocopies in a safe place. If you're covered by a secondary insurer, you'll need to make two photocopies of the bill, one for your records and one for the secondary insurer. That may save you a great deal of time later on, if a bill is lost or misplaced.

In addition, if you are filing a claim for a significant amount of money, it's usually best to file it separately, without attaching other medical bills to the claim form. Filing a large group of bills at the same time—with a single claim form—may seem easier, but it may also increase the likelihood that bills may be misplaced or processed incorrectly.

Another important advantage of attaching only one medical bill to each claim form is that it makes it much easier to understand the Explanation of Benefits Statement from the insurer, and to quickly identify any claim-processing errors. If you file a group of claims, the EOBS may include all the payments together as if they represented a single bill.

For example, I once sent eight bills to an insurer with a single claim form. All of the bills were for prescription medications, and they totaled $600. The insurance policy I had at that time provided reimbursement for prescription medications at the 80% rate (an 80/20 plan) under major medical. I knew that

I had already met the deductible for the year, and I therefore expected $480 in reimbursement. The insurance company check, however, was for less than $400.

Since I had sent the bills in together, attached to a single claim form, the EOBS listed only the total amount of the claim and the reimbursement amount. There was no indication of which bills were paid and which were not. Under the section labeled "Provider" on the EOBS, it just said "Prescriptions." It took almost an hour on the telephone with an insurance company representative to review the bills individually and to make sense of the reimbursement provided by the insurer.

Fortunately, it turned out to be a simple error. The insurer had mistakenly decided that two of the bills were duplicates and had paid only seven bills instead of eight. Although I eventually received full reimbursement for the eighth bill, sorting out the problem required a great deal of work. If I had sent the bills in individually—a few days apart—with a separate claim form for each bill, they would have been processed separately. I would then have received a separate EOBS for each claim, and I would have been able to identify the error immediately.

STEP FOUR: SETTING UP A RECORD KEEPING SYSTEM

Setting up and maintaining a record keeping system is an essential part of ensuring that you obtain the health insurance benefits to which you are entitled. Before sending in a claim, record the name of the medical provider, the date of service, the amount of the bill, the type of treatment or test, and the date you're mailing in the claim on a record keeping form (See Table 9). Record an estimate of the amount of reimbursement that you expect from the insurance company, as well, based on your understanding of your health insurance policy.

Writing down that estimate before mailing the claim to the insurer is a good way to test your understanding of the policy rules and to establish a basis for reviewing the insurance company's reimbursement. When you eventually receive the

EOBS from your insurer, note the amount of the actual reimbursement below your estimate on the record keeping form. If you're unsure of what claims have been included in the EOBS, call the company and review the details.

Although you may occasionally make an error, in the overwhelming majority of cases you should be able to accurately estimate the amount of reimbursement that will be provided by your insurer. If you find that your estimates are frequently inaccurate, you may need to review your information file to make certain that you've understood the policy rules. If your estimates are accurate, and your insurer has made an error in processing your claim, you will need to file a claim appeal to ensure that you receive the appropriate benefits. (See Step Five for a discussion of the procedures involved in filing a claim appeal.)

It's essential to compare your estimate of the insurance company reimbursement with the actual reimbursement each time you receive an Explanation of Benefits Statement. It's sort of like balancing a checking account. You can probably get by without balancing your checking account for a while—at least until the bank begins to charge you for overdrawn checks—but you'll save a lot of money by balancing the account on a regular basis. In the same way, regularly comparing your estimates with the actual amount of reimbursement provided by your insurer is likely to lead to significant savings and to a better understanding of the policy rules.

You can maintain records of your medical claims in a notebook, on sheets of paper, or on index cards. If you have a computer, you can use a database program to record information about your health insurance claims, as well. In addition to recording basic information, it's also important to include a section called "Completed" on your record form. When you first create a record for a new claim, enter "no" in that section. When the claim has been paid in accordance with the policy rules, change the "no" to a "yes."

Table 9
Sample Record Keeping Form

Medical Provider	
Date of Service	
Type of Treatment or Test	
Amount of Bill	
Date Claim Filed with Insurer	
Estimate of Reimbursement	
Actual Reimbursement	
Date Reimbursement Received	
Completed	
Notes (Deductible, Co-Payments)	

Table 9 is designed for a situation in which an individual is covered by a single insurer. If you have both a primary and a secondary insurer, you'll need to include additional spaces to record information concerning reimbursements from your secondary insurer.

Be sure to also note information in your records about the amount of the deductible that has been met at each point. That will help you maintain up-to-date information in regard to the yearly deductible, so that you'll know when the individual and the family deductible have been met in full.

Review your records periodically. Note those records that have a "no" in the "Completed" field and that are more than five weeks old (many insurance companies process claims in three to four weeks). If there are records in that group that your insurer does not appear to have processed, file the claim again. Include a photocopy of the original bill and a new claim form. Write "Second Request" on the top of the claim form. If you don't receive a response within four weeks, file a formal claim appeal (See Step Five).

STEP FIVE: DEVELOPING A METHOD FOR FILING CLAIM APPEALS

A **claim appeal** is a request that an insurer review a specific claim and the level of reimbursement provided for possible errors. Claim appeals play a very important role in ensuring that health insurance benefits are paid appropriately, and they represent an important part of this six-step approach to developing a systematic method for dealing with claims.

Many people have reported that although they sometimes feel that their insurance company may have made an error in processing their claims, they are anxious about filing an appeal. Although that's understandable—it can be somewhat frightening to question a decision made by a large organization—the anxiety is unnecessary. Questions about coverage, the meaning of particular policy rules, and reimbursement amounts are not unusual in the health insurance field, and are generally dealt with by insurers in a highly professional manner. As long as your appeal is presented in a calm, reasonable way, the insurer will generally respond on a similar level.

If you have never filed a claim appeal and are anxious about doing so, the easiest way to deal with that anxiety is to set up a standardized claim appeal form. In addition to helping to reduce anxiety, developing a standardized claim appeal form also saves time and ensures that you won't forget to include important information when you file an appeal.

Your claim appeal form should include your insurance company identification number, prominently displayed near the top of the form. It should also include the name of the policyholder (the insured)—if different than the patient—the name of the patient, and the patient's address and telephone number. There should also be spaces labeled, "Provider," "Date of

Service," and so on, where you can fill in the appropriate information (See Table 10).

Include several lines at the bottom, as well, labeled "Please Note." In that section, you can describe the problem you're experiencing from your point of view. For example, if the claim was rejected by error on the grounds that it was a duplicate of an earlier claim, you can briefly explain the differences between the two claims.

It's important to keep your explanation brief, clear, and unemotional, even though you may be upset with the situation. The clearer and simpler the explanation, the more likely that your request will be clearly understood and that the error will be corrected quickly. If you're not certain what to write in the "Please Note" section, you can print a general statement such as, "Please review this claim."

Print or type the information on the claim appeal form to make certain that it's clearly legible. To save time, you can fill out the basic information—the policyholder's name and insurance company identification number, your address, and so on—and then photocopy the form. When you're ready to file a claim appeal, you'll only have to fill out the information related to the provider, the date of service, and a description of the problem.

Do not include information on the claim appeal form about problems that are not directly related to the immediate issue, and don't include comments about your general experiences with the insurance company. Including irrelevant information about issues that are not directly related to the immediate problem may confuse the situation and thus delay the appeals process.

If additional documentation—a letter from your doctor explaining the medical need for a specific treatment or procedure or for particular medical equipment, an operative report, a copy of an itemized hospital bill—appears to be required, also include that material with your claim appeal. Note the fact that the documentation is attached to the claim appeal form in the "Documentation Attached" section.

Table 10
Sample Claim Appeal Form

Claim Appeal

Identification #_____
Name of Policyholder_____
Name of Patient_____
Address_____
City _____ State/ZIP code_____
Telephone_____
Provider_____
Date of Service_____
Please Note_____

_____
Documentation Attached_____

If you're going to attach a doctor's letter to the claim appeal form, it's helpful if all related background information is included in that letter. Although the insurance company may have detailed records of your illnesses and your medical history, it may speed up the appeals process if a summary of that information—certified by a doctor's letter—is included with each claim appeal that includes a letter from a medical provider. Insurers deal with thousands of claims, and the person evaluating your claim appeal may not necessarily be aware of the details of your diagnosis or your medical history.

If you're uncertain what information or documentation should be included with your claim appeal, call the insurance company and discuss the situation with a company representative. However, it's important to be aware that in some insurance companies, the people who answer the telephones may not be expected to provide detailed information or to fully explain insurance company policies.

If that's the way your insurance company is organized, ask to speak with a supervisor. Supervisors have generally worked at the company for a long time, and are usually very knowledgeable about policy rules. If you call your insurer to discuss a claim problem, and you find a particularly helpful supervisor, ask if you can mail or fax your claim appeal directly to that person. For future reference, include the supervisor's name, telephone number, and fax number in your information file, as well.

Claim appeals should always be made in writing, so that there's a record of the appeal. They should also generally be sent to the insurance company by certified mail, with return receipt requested, so that you have a record that the appeal was received by the insurer. In addition, the envelope in which the claim appeal is sent should have the words "Claim Appeal" written in large letters in the address to make certain that the appeal is forwarded to the correct department. Be certain also to include a copy of the original medical bill and the EOBS with your claim appeal. Keep a copy of all of the documents that you send to your insurer for your own records, of course. Following these procedures will help ensure that your claim appeal will be reviewed as quickly as possible.

STEP SIX: ESTABLISHING A SYSTEM FOR REQUESTING HELP FROM GOVERNMENT AGENCIES OR PRIVATE ORGANIZATIONS

Claim-processing problems may result from communications difficulties or data entry errors, or from difficulties in understanding an insurer's requirements for specific information or documentation. Such difficulties can often be resolved in a satisfactory manner through the appeals process.

However, there are times when an insurer and a consumer may disagree on the interpretation or application of specific health insurance policy rules or state or federal laws or regulations. Where significant amounts of money are involved, or where a specific principle is at issue, it's often important for consumers to request help from private, state, or federal agencies or organizations in resolving a particular problem.

The first step in the process is to try to determine the organization or agency to which your request for help should be addressed. Addressing the request to the wrong group simply delays the matter. The most important factor in deciding which organization or agency to contact has to do with whether the issue relates primarily to state or to federal laws or regulations. Unfortunately, given the chaotic nature of the current health insurance system, that's not always easy for a consumer to determine.

Your request for help should probably be addressed to a state agency rather than to a federal agency if the problem has to do with the way in which a traditional individual or group insurer or a managed care program

- has processed a claim;
- has determined the level of reimbursement in reference to a claim;
- has interpreted a specific state law or regulation or a health insurance policy rule in a manner with which you disagree.

On the state level, you can write to your state Department of Insurance or Department of Health for help. Although the structure differs from state to state, in some states the Department of Insurance deals with situations related to traditional insurers while the Department of Health deals with situations related to managed care plans or hospitals. Some states also have separate insurance boards that deal with specific aspects of health insurance, such as individual or small employer insurance plans. Check with your state Department of Insurance to determine the specific structure in your state.

In some areas, the local county or state medical society may also help solve specific health insurance claim problems related to medical bills from doctors, testing centers, or hospitals. Check with your county or state medical society to determine if a program exists in your area. (See Chapter 6 for a further discussion of claim appeals related to self-funded plans. See Chapter 7 for a further discussion of claim appeals related to managed care plans.)

Your request for help should probably be addressed to a federal agency rather than to a state agency if the claim problem appears to relate to an issue in regard to which the federal government has passed a specific law. At this point, federal laws deal with a number of health insurance issues, including

- coverage for pregnancy and childbirth;
- yearly or lifetime benefit maximums for the treatment of mental or emotional illnesses;
- transfers from one group health insurance plan to another;
- extensions of group health insurance after divorce or after leaving a job;
- coverage under a self-funded plan;
- discrimination on the basis of disability;
- issues related to Medicare, Medicare HMOs, Medigap policies, CHAMPUS, or Medical Savings Accounts.

If the issue relates to a specific federal law or regulation, you'll also need to identify the appropriate federal agency. Issues that involve self-funded plans or extensions of private group health insurance plans under COBRA should be directed to the Pension and Welfare Benefits Administration of the United States Department of Labor. Issues that involve extensions under COBRA of health insurance plans sponsored by state or municipal government agencies should be directed to the United States Public Health Service. (See Appendix B for information on how to contact these agencies.)

At times, a particular health insurance issue may relate to both state and federal laws or regulations. In such cases, it's generally best to begin on the state level. If state agencies or organizations are unable to help resolve the problem, you can then turn to federal agencies for help.

Once you've identified the appropriate state or federal agency or organization, the second step is to formulate a letter that is likely to result in a successful resolution of the problem. Your letter should be unemotional, highly factual, and very specific. It should focus on the immediate issue, and should not include a discussion of other issues that are not directly related. In addition, it should refer to the specific parts of your health insurance policy or to the specific state or federal laws or regulations that you believe may have been misinterpreted or incorrectly applied. If you're not certain which regulations are involved, you can keep the letter very general. However, the more specific you are the more likely it is that your request for help will be processed quickly.

Attach the appropriate documentation to your letter, including copies of all related medical bills, a letter from your doctor explaining the need for the treatment or service, copies of letters and Explanation of Benefits Statements you've received from your insurer, and photocopies of relevant sections of your health insurance policy. Your medical provider, the local medical society, or a representative of your state Department of Insurance may be able to help you phrase the letter effectively, and may also be able to help you determine what documentation should be included.

Make certain that you keep a copy of the letter and of all related documentation. If you don't receive a response within thirty days, follow up with another letter. Note in that letter that this is your second request. Include a copy of your first letter and the related documentation, just in case the paperwork has been lost or misplaced.

If following these steps does not lead to a resolution of the problem, you have several additional choices. One possibility is to talk with a private medical claim-processing company. For years, many doctors and hospitals have employed claim-processing companies to file claims or to deal with problems related to claim-processing. Over the past few years, many of those companies have begun to work for consumers, as well, helping to solve claim-processing problems.

At this point, there are no national licensing requirements for private medical claim-processors, and there are no national rules or regulations in terms of procedures or charges. Each medical claim-processing company has its own approach to dealing with claims, and charges vary from company to company. Some medical claim-processing companies charge a flat monthly fee for processing claims. Other companies charge an hourly fee, and others charge on the basis of a percentage of the total claim.

You may be able to locate a medical claim-processing company by looking in the telephone book or in your local newspaper. The **National Association of Claims Assistance Professionals** (**NACAP**), which has 1,500 members at present, can also help you locate a medical claim-processing company in your area (See Appendix B). Some members of NACAP focus primarily on claim-processing for medical providers. Other claim-processing companies work with both medical providers and consumers, or with consumers only.

You can also discuss health insurance problems with a private organization. (See Chapter 9 for information on private organizations that offer help with Medicare-related problems.) You can consult an attorney, as well, to determine whether legal issues may be involved in a particular health insurance problem. As we discussed earlier, there are an enormous number of state and federal laws and regulations that relate to health insurance. An attorney can review those laws and regulations with you, and can determine whether they may relate to your particular problem.

If your health insurance problem appears to be shared by many other individuals, you may also be able to enlist the help of your state or federal legislative representatives. Neither the state nor the federal legislature generally has any direct influence on specific decisions related to individual health insurance problems, even if those problems involve a government-sponsored program such as CHAMPUS, COBRA, Medicare, Medicaid, or ERISA. However, legislative representatives can schedule hearings to deal with general health insurance issues, and can consider the possibility of introducing new legislation to deal with problems that affect a large number of people. In fact, many of the new state and federal health insurance laws that now help to protect the rights of consumers were passed because of support from citizens who had experienced specific health insurance problems.

The likelihood that the state or federal legislature will focus on a particular type of health insurance problem may increase with the number of letters that legislators receive on the issue. One way to help ensure that legislators will consider specific health insurance issues is to join an existing advocacy or self-help group that deals with those issues, or to form a new advocacy group to deal with specific concerns. (See the listing for the **American Self-Help Clearinghouse** in Appendix B for information about existing advocacy and self-help groups.)

SUMMARY

In order to obtain maximum benefits from your health insurance policy, it's essential to develop a systematic approach to dealing with health insurance claims. The six-step approach suggested in this chapter includes

- setting up an information file;
- using the predetermination of benefits process;
- establishing an efficient claim-filing system;
- setting up an effective record keeping system;
- developing a method for filing claim appeals with your insurer;
- establishing a system for requesting help from private organizations and state or federal agencies.

In many cases, following those steps will help to prevent health insurance problems from occurring, or will help to quickly resolve those problems that do occur. However, if those steps do not lead to a resolution of a specific problem, you can request help from a private medical claim-processing company, the state or local medical society, an attorney, or your state or federal legislative representatives.

Although some people may feel anxious about questioning the decisions of an insurance company—or of any large organization—filing appeals when appropriate is essential to making certain that you obtain the health insurance benefits to which you're entitled. As long as a claim appeal is presented in a calm, reasonable way, insurers will generally respond in a similar manner, thus allowing the problem to be resolved.

Once you've understood the technical terms and phrases used in the health insurance field and the overall structure of the current system, and once you've developed a systematic approach to dealing with claims, you have the basic tools you need to deal effectively with your health insurance problems.

Part II
HEALTH INSURANCE PLANS

4

Traditional Individual and Group Plans, Doctors' Bills

Although individuals don't generally sign formal contracts with insurance companies, an insurance policy nevertheless represents an agreement. In the case of an individual health insurance policy, the agreement is between the consumer and the insurance company; in the case of an employer-sponsored group health insurance plan, the agreement is between the employer and the insurance company.

The principle is the same in both cases: The individual or the employer pays a monthly or quarterly premium to the insurance company, and the insurer provides reimbursement for the individual's claims—and for the claims of other participants in the case of a group plan—for specific medical treatments, tests, and services. Coverage for such treatments, tests, and services under a health insurance policy is always limited and is always subject to detailed policy rules.

REVIEWING POLICY RULES

Given the cost of medical care, your health insurance policy represents one of the most important agreements with which you'll ever be involved. Thus, it's essential that you understand the policy rules in detail. Unfortunately, there's often a great deal of misunderstanding and miscommunication between insurance companies and consumers in regard to health insurance policy rules. The problem is compounded by the fact that insurance policies are not generally standardized. In fact, they often vary a great deal in terms of the treatments and services that are covered, and in terms of the rules under which the policy operates. Furthermore, policy provisions are often complex, and the state and federal regulations that govern health insurance are often difficult to comprehend. However, in spite of those difficulties, it's essential that you try to understand your health insurance policy so that you can obtain the maximum benefits to which you're entitled.

In order to understand a health insurance policy, you need to carefully read the policy itself. The best time to do that is before a problem arises, so that you'll have time to fully understand the policy provisions. Reading the policy booklet offers an overall view of the policy and may be sufficient for most situations. However, in some cases the booklets that are issued to consumers may represent only a summary of the policy provisions. A full description of those provisions may be found in the full contract.

If you have concerns about coverage for specific treatments, tests, or services, it may be helpful to read the related sections of the full contract. In the case of an individual policy, a copy of the contract or a detailed explanation of specific contract provisions may be available from the insurer. In the case of an employer-sponsored group health insurance plan, the relevant parts of the **master contract**—the agreement between the employer and the insurer—may be available from the employer's benefits manager.

The master contract for a group health insurance plan is often highly technical and may be quite lengthy. You may only need a copy of certain sections. If you're unable to obtain a copy of those sections, either your employer's benefits manager or the insurer may be able to provide a detailed summary of specific provisions or may be able to offer answers to questions about particular benefits.

Once you've reviewed the contract, you're ready to begin to deal with any problems that might develop. In this chapter, we will discuss the types of problems that may occur in relation to claims filed with individual and group health insurance plans for doctors' bills. Chapter 5 will review the types of problems that may occur in relation to hospital bills. This chapter and Chapter 5 will also include a discussion of possible solutions to specific problems.

PROBLEMS WITH THE YEARLY DEDUCTIBLE

In theory, keeping track of the yearly major medical deductible—the amount you need to pay each year before the insurer begins to provide reimbursement for major medical claims—should be simple. In reality, it seems to represent one of the most common sources of confusion for consumers. There are two difficulties. First, insurance companies don't necessarily subtract the deductible from the first major medical claim of the year. In fact, in some cases, a number of claims may be processed before the deductible is subtracted.

Second, certain medical tests such as X-rays and blood tests may be covered under the basic benefits provision of the policy, and reimbursement may therefore be provided by the insurer even though the deductible has not yet been met. As a result, you may find that a number of bills are paid in full at the beginning of the year even though the deductible has not been subtracted.

As difficult as it may be to keep track of the deductible under those conditions, it's important to do so. One of the advantages of using the record keeping system discussed earlier is that the system makes it easy to keep track of the deductible. Using that record keeping system will help to ensure that you are always aware of the point at which the deductible has been met for the year.

PROBLEMS RELATED TO PROCEDURE CODES

Many consumers report that there are times when the reimbursement that their insurers offer is far lower than the actual medical bill, and that they are thus sometimes obligated to pay large **balance bills.** A balance bill is the difference between the provider's bill and the amount of reimbursement offered by the insurance company.

A large balance bill may result from a number of factors. One possible reason for a large balance bill is that the provider's bill may have contained an error, particularly in terms of the **procedure code.** Every medical treatment, test, or service has a specific procedure code. Insurers generally process claims on the basis of those codes. If the code listed on a medical bill is incorrect, it may result in a far lower level of reimbursement. Since a procedure code error is fairly easy to correct—the provider's office can check the procedure code by reviewing the chart—that's the first area to examine whenever the amount of reimbursement provided by an insurance company appears to be too low.

PROBLEMS RELATED TO THE UCR

If the procedure code is listed correctly, then the balance bill may be a result of the difference between the Usual and Customary Rate (the UCR)—as determined by the insurer—and the provider's charge. Insurers generally determine the UCR through a statistical analysis of providers' charges in a specific geographic area. Some insurance companies develop their own UCR database, while other insurers may use a database provided by another company. Thus, the UCR for a particular procedure may not be identical from insurer to insurer, or from one geographic area to another.

The UCR represents the maximum amount of reimbursement an insurer will generally consider for a particular test or procedure. Medical providers are not obligated to limit their bills to an insurer's determination of the UCR, and patients are generally considered to be responsible for the entire bill, even if there's a large difference between the bill and the reimbursement provided by the insurance company.

For example, let's assume that you've met the deductible for the year but have not yet met the yearly co-payment maximum. Your health insurance policy provides for payment of major medical claims at the 80% rate (an 80/20 plan), and you have filed a claim for a $100 doctor's bill that was related to an office visit. If the UCR for the office visit is $100, you'll generally receive $80 (80% of the bill), leaving you responsible for paying the $20 balance (the co-payment or co-insurance).

However, if the UCR is only $85, the insurer will view that amount as the maximum it will consider in terms of reimbursement, rather than the $100 amount of the bill itself. In that case, the maximum reimbursement the insurer will provide will be $68 (80% of $85), and you will be responsible for paying the remaining $32. That $32 includes the $17 co-payment and the $15 that the insurer considered to be above the UCR.

The percentile that your insurer uses to determine the UCR may also have a significant effect on reimbursement. (See "Problems Related to Percentiles," below.)

In some cases, once an insurer has determined the UCR, there may not be a great deal you can do to change that determination. Many insurers appear to consider their UCR analyses—and the database on which those analyses are based—to be private information, and they seem to be reluctant to share that information with consumers. That obviously makes it difficult for a consumer to review the way in which the database has been established or the process that was used to determine the UCR.

Because of that difficulty, it's usually better to try to prevent such situations from occurring whenever possible by using the predetermination of benefits process in advance of treatment in all non-emergency situations that involve significant costs (See Chapter 3). If it's not possible to use the predetermination of benefits process prior to treatment, and the eventual reimbursement provided by your insurer turns out to be far lower than the provider's bill, there are several steps you can take that may be helpful in some cases.

One approach is to ask the insurer to make certain that the ZIP code used for the UCR analysis is correct. Since a UCR analysis is generally based on a database of statistical information related to providers' charges in a particular geographic area, the ZIP code that's used for the analysis is often very important. At times, errors may occur in terms of selecting the correct ZIP code. Such errors may be the result of a simple data entry error in which an incorrect ZIP code is unintentionally entered into the computer, or may result from confusion caused by a situation in which a doctor may have more than one office or may work out of both an office and a hospital.

In the latter case, it's important to make certain that the correct address—the address of the office or hospital where the treatment was actually performed—is used as the basis for the UCR analysis. For example, a few years ago I helped a reader deal with a problem involving a claim for approximately $1,200 for an outpatient procedure that had been performed at a local hospital. The insurance company provided less than $800 as reimbursement, leaving a balance bill of more than $400.

Although the doctor worked at the hospital, he also had two separate offices outside of the hospital. The address of each of those offices was printed on the bill that was submitted to the insurance company. The office in which the patient had originally been examined was near the hospital; the doctor's other office was farther away, in another town.

By error, the insurance company had used the address of the office farthest from the hospital as the basis for the UCR analysis, even though the original exam had taken place at the office nearest the hospital and the procedure had taken place at the hospital itself. I asked a supervisor at the insurance company to review the UCR, using either the hospital address (where the treatment had occurred) or the address of the doctor's office nearest the hospital (where the patient had originally been examined). Both were in the same ZIP code. When the analysis was redone, the amount of reimbursement was increased by more than $300, leaving a balance of less than $100.

If the ZIP code that the insurer used to determine the UCR

is correct in a particular case, the next step is to talk with your medical provider about how his fees compare to those of other local providers, and to check with the local medical society to try to determine a range of bills for the procedure from other providers in the area. If your doctor's fee is similar to, or lower than, the fees of other providers in the area for the same procedure, you can send in a claim appeal asking the insurer to review the UCR analysis. Include the information provided by your doctor and the local medical society with your appeal. That may be sufficient to persuade your insurer to reconsider the UCR determination.

In some cases, that claim appeal may lead to a successful resolution of the problem. If it does not, the next step is to write to your county or state medical society or to your state Department of Insurance and ask for their help. (See Chapter 3 for more information on claim appeals.)

PROBLEMS RELATED TO PERCENTILES

The **percentile system** may directly affect the determination of the UCR. However, the system is complex, and involves a number of highly technical issues. A percentile and a percent are quite different. In non-technical terms, a percentile—as it's used in the health insurance field—refers to the level at which a particular percentage of charges falls for a specific procedure in a geographic area.

A full analysis of the basis for the reimbursement provided for a specific treatment requires information about the database used by the insurer and about the percentile used to determine the UCR. Insurers do not generally share detailed information about the database with consumers. However, the general principle is simple as it relates to the percentile: The lower the percentile, the lower the amount of reimbursement that's likely to be provided for major medical claims.

Let's assume that your policy provides for payment of major medical claims at the 80% rate (an 80/20 plan), that you have met the yearly deductible but have not yet met the yearly co-payment maximum, and that you have filed a $1,000 major medical claim. That would generally allow for a maximum possible reimbursement of $800 (80% of $1,000), leaving a balance of $200. If your insurer sets payments to the ninetieth percentile, reimbursement will probably be provided for the full $800 in the majority of cases. However, if your insurer sets payments to the fiftieth, sixtieth, seventieth or eightieth percentile, reimbursement may be a great deal lower.

Table 11 contains an array of charges for the treatment of an appendectomy, the surgical removal of an appendix. As an illustration of the percentile system, let's assume that the surgeon's charge for the appendectomy was $1,600. Since Table 11 is intended to serve as an illustration of the basic concepts, neither the amount of the surgeon's charge nor the figures in the table represent actual amounts.

In this case, if the insurer sets reimbursement to the fiftieth percentile, the maximum amount that the insurer would consider for the appendectomy would be $1,000. If the insurance policy provides reimbursement of major medical bills at the 80% rate (an 80/20 plan), and the surgeon's bill is $1,600, the actual reimbursement would be $800 (80% of $1,000), leaving a balance bill of $800.

However, if the insurer sets reimbursement to the eightieth percentile in this case, the company would consider a maximum of $1,300. In that case, the actual reimbursement would be $1,040 (80% of $1,300), leaving a balance bill of $560. If the insurer sets reimbursement to the ninetieth percentile, the insurer would consider a maximum of $1,650. That would be reduced to $1,600, the amount of the bill. In that case, the actual reimbursement would be $1,280 (80% of $1,600). That would leave a balance bill of only $320. Thus, the percentile that's used by an insurer in determining the UCR may significantly affect the amount of reimbursement (See Table 11).

The percentile system may not always be discussed in detail in health insurance policy booklets. You may need to check with your insurer to determine the specific percentile that is used by the company.

Table 11
Hypothetical Example of Charges and Percentiles for an Appendectomy

| | Percentile | | | |
	50th	60th	70th	80th
Charge	$1,000	$1,100	$1,200	$1,300

| | Percentile | | |
	85th	90th	95th
Charge	$1,400	$1,650	$1,800

PROBLEMS RELATED TO CHILDBIRTH AND PREGNANCY

Over the past few years, one of the major issues in the health insurance field has revolved around the number of days of hospital care that should be covered by a health insurance policy for childbirth. Many people have felt strongly that the standard hospital stay for childbirth should be at least 48 hours. A number of state legislatures have discussed the issue, and several states have passed legislation to require insurers that offer coverage for childbirth to provide coverage for a full 48 hours in the hospital. However, state laws that relate to benefits apply only to health insurance policies within the particular state, and do not generally apply to self-funded plans, since such plans are regulated through federal law rather than through state laws.

In order to deal with this issue on a national basis, the federal government passed the **Newborns' and Mothers' Health Protection Act** in the fall of 1996. The act is effective as of January 1, 1998. Although it does not require insurers to provide coverage for childbirth, the Newborns' and Mothers' Health Protection Act does require that health insurance policies and self-funded plans that do offer such coverage must provide benefits for a full 48 hours of hospital care following childbirth, and 96 hours of hospital care following a Caesarean delivery. However, in certain situations state law may take precedence in terms of health insurance coverage for childbirth, particularly if the state has passed a law providing for similar requirements.

In addition, the **Portability and Accountability Act**—passed in 1996—provides that group health insurance plans may not generally consider pregnancy to be a pre-existing condition. That provision becomes effective as group plans are first renewed after July 1, 1997.

PROBLEMS RELATED TO CLAIMS FOR PSYCHOLOGICAL OR PSYCHIATRIC TREATMENT

In many health insurance policies, there may be a significant difference between the reimbursement provided for the treatment of illnesses such as cancer or heart disease and the reimbursement provided for the treatment of mental or emotional illnesses. That difference is generally referred to as a **lack of parity.** It can obviously have serious economic consequences for individuals who need treatment for a mental or emotional illness.

A guarantee of parity was included in one of the original proposals for the federal Portability and Accountability Act. Although the act was passed in the summer of 1996, the guarantee of parity—which would have ensured full equality of benefits in terms of reimbursement for the treatment of both physical and mental illnesses—was not included in the final version.

However, the federal **Mental Health Parity Act,** passed in October of 1996, focused on this issue once again. The act specifically prohibits insurers that offer coverage for the treatment of mental illnesses from establishing lower yearly or lifetime benefit maximums for reimbursement for the treatment of mental illness than for the treatment of physical illness.

The act does not guarantee full parity, though, and it does not require insurers to provide coverage for the treatment of mental illnesses. Nor does the act prohibit insurers from including other differences in benefits between reimbursement for the treatment of mental and physical illness. It refers only to yearly and lifetime benefit maximums.

In addition, there are some specific exclusions. First, the act applies only to group insurance plans sponsored by companies that have more than fifty employees. Thus, it does not directly affect individual or small group health insurance policies. Second, if a company can demonstrate that the act results in increased costs of 1% or more, the company may be exempt from the act's requirements. Although those limitations may pose serious problems in some cases, the Mental Health Parity Act nevertheless represents an important step forward.

The Mental Health Parity Act is effective as of January of 1998. Hopefully, it will help to prevent the severe economic difficulties that some people who need treatment for mental illnesses have experienced in the past when they reached the yearly or lifetime benefit maximums.

A number of states have also passed laws dealing with mental health parity. Although those laws may refer to many health insurance policies offered within the particular state, they do not generally affect self-funded plans. The laws differ significantly from state to state. Check with your state Department of Insurance or with NAMI (the National Alliance for the Mentally Ill) to determine whether your state currently has a law that affects parity (See Appendix B).

PROBLEMS RELATED TO SECONDARY INSURANCE

Secondary insurance may be available whenever two individuals in a family each have separate health insurance policies that provide for family coverage. The process of determining such benefits is often referred to as the **coordination-of-benefits** system. Secondary insurance benefits may provide a significant amount of reimbursement—particularly for families with high medical bills—and can thus be important from an economic point of view.

However, there are a number of problems that may occur when dealing with secondary coverage. One of the most common problems has to do with trying to determine which insurance policy is primary and which is secondary, particularly when the claim is for a child. That determination is important, since claims must be sent first to the child's primary insurer. Once the primary insurer has paid its portion of the bill, the claim can be submitted to the secondary insurer.

Until a few years ago, it was often assumed that a father's health insurance policy represented a child's primary insurer. However, these days, if both parents have health insurance policies that provide for family coverage, the primary status is often assigned to the parent whose birth date comes earlier in the year.

Thus, if a child's mother was born in September, and the child's father was born in October, the mother's insurance policy would generally be considered the child's primary insurer and the father's policy would be considered the secondary insurer. The determination of which parent's insurance policy is primary for a child in a situation in which both parents have health insurance with family coverage generally depends only on the month and date of the parents' birth, not on the year in which the parents were born. Check with your insurance company to review their system for determining the primary insurer in such situations.

Once the primary insurer has been determined, the next step is to make certain that you understand the coordination-of-benefits system that your insurer uses to determine secondary benefits. In some insurance policies, the secondary benefits system provides for reimbursement of up to 80% for covered medical expenses. Those benefits, of course, apply only to that portion of the bill for which reimbursement was not provided by the primary insurer.

For example, let's assume that both parents have separate health insurance policies with family coverage, and that both policies pay 80% of all covered major medical claims in terms of both primary and secondary benefits. Assume as well that the family deductible has already been met for the year in both policies, and that the mother's insurance policy is primary for the children, since her birth date comes earlier in the year than the father's.

If the mother files a claim for her child for $100 with her insurer, and if that amount is within the UCR, her policy will provide $80 in reimbursement (80% of $100). If the father's policy pays secondary insurance benefits at the 80% rate, his policy will provide $16 in reimbursement (80% of the remaining $20), leaving a balance of only $4.

However, some insurance policies may include very different rules in relation to coordination-of-benefits. For example, in some cases reimbursement may be provided at the 50%, 60%, or 70% rate, rather than at the 80% rate. In other cases, secondary insurance benefits may apply to children who are covered by their parents' health insurance policies but may not apply to the parents if they are both covered by the same health insurance plan. For that reason, it's important to make certain that you understand your policy's provisions in terms of secondary insurance benefits.

CLAIM DENIALS ON THE GROUNDS THAT A TREATMENT IS NOT A COVERED EXPENSE

Certain treatments and services are specifically excluded by many health insurance policies. Claims for such treatments are generally denied on the grounds that they do not represent a covered expense or that they are not medically necessary under the terms of the policy. For example, many traditional individual and group policies may specifically exclude expenses related to cosmetic surgery, hearing aids, or eyeglasses.

Insurance companies want to be certain that services and treatments that are specifically excluded by a policy are not paid for by error. Thus, an insurer may occasionally request additional information or documentation before providing reimbursement for a claim that appears as if it is related to such excluded services or treatments. Thus, if your insurance policy excludes coverage for eyeglasses, your insurance company may request additional information if you file a claim that relates to medical treatment that appears to involve related eye problems. In the same way, if your insurance policy specifically excludes coverage for cosmetic surgery—as many health insurance policies do—your insurer may request additional information before processing a claim related to surgery of the face or nose.

In such cases, if the claim is for an expense that should be covered under the policy, all that's generally needed is to file a claim appeal that includes a letter from your doctor explaining the specific medical need for the treatment. If the treatment involved surgery, include a copy of the operative report and a copy of the hospital bill with the claim appeal. You can obtain a copy of the operative report from your surgeon, and you can obtain a copy of the hospital bill from the hospital billing office.

CLAIM DENIALS ON THE GROUNDS THAT A TREATMENT IS NOT MEDICALLY NECESSARY

As we discussed earlier, some insurance companies seem to use the phrase "not medically necessary" in two different ways. In some cases, the phrase may be used to mean that the company needs additional information or documentation before it can determine whether or not a claim is eligible for coverage. In other cases, the phrase may be used to mean that the insurer has concluded that the claim is not eligible for coverage under the terms of the policy. In the former case, it would seem to make sense for the insurance company to be as specific as possible in terms of the information or documentation that's needed. However, instead of listing the specific documentation that's required, at times some insurance companies limit their explanations to the phrase "not medically necessary."

If a claim is denied on the grounds that the treatment or service is not medically necessary, and you believe that the claim should be covered by your policy, try to determine how the phrase is being used. If the insurer is requesting additional information or documentation before making a decision about the medical necessity of the treatment, you need to determine the specific documentation that the company requires. If the answer is not obvious from the EOBS, call the company and discuss the issue with a representative. Once you have determined what documentation is needed—a letter from your doctor, a copy of an operative report, a copy of an itemized hospital bill—file an immediate claim appeal that includes the required material.

If the insurer is using the phrase to mean that it has concluded that the treatment does not meet the requirement of medical necessity under the terms of the policy and is thus not covered, and you are convinced that the claim should be covered, ask your doctor to write a letter explaining the medical need for the treatment. Then file a claim appeal that includes the doctor's letter.

PROBLEMS RELATED TO COVERAGE FOR DURABLE MEDICAL EQUIPMENT

In some cases, claims for durable medical equipment—braces, crutches, wheelchairs—that should be covered by an insurance policy may be denied simply because they are not yet on the insurance company's list of "medically necessary equipment." In such cases, the Explanation of Benefits Statement may include a note that the equipment is not a covered expense or is not medically necessary.

For example, when I first began to use a power wheelchair, I anticipated that I might have some difficulty obtaining reimbursement from my insurance company. Power wheelchairs, after all, are quite expensive. My first power wheelchair cost more than $6,000. However, the claim was approved without any problem. A year and a half later, I bought new batteries for the chair. I filed a claim, and I attached a copy of the bill and a letter from my doctor explaining the need for the batteries.

Although the batteries were only $200, both the claim and the initial claim appeal I filed were rejected with the explanation that the batteries were not medically necessary and did not represent a covered expense. After several telephone calls to a supervisor at my insurance company, I discovered the problem: power wheelchairs were on the insurance company's list of medically necessary equipment, but wheelchair batteries were not.

I wrote a letter to the insurer, asking that the company review the question of whether wheelchair batteries should be added to the company's list of medically necessary equipment. I waited a month and filed another claim appeal. A few weeks later, I received a check from the insurer for the cost of the batteries.

If a claim for medical equipment is denied, talk with an insurance company representative to determine whether the equipment is on the insurer's list of medically necessary items. If it is not on that list, and you think it should be covered by the policy, write and ask the company to consider adding it. Then, wait a few weeks and file a claim appeal.

CLAIM DENIALS ON THE GROUNDS THAT THE TREATMENT IS EXPERIMENTAL

Claims may occasionally be denied on the grounds that a particular treatment or test is experimental. My experience suggests that there may be times when a new treatment or test is viewed as standard medical practice by a provider, but may be viewed as experimental under the terms of some insurance policies. In some cases, a claim appeal that includes a letter from a provider or from the local medical society specifying that the treatment or test is considered standard medical practice—assuming that is the case—may be sufficient to persuade an insurance company to review it's earlier determination.

However, it's important to remember that reimbursement is generally based on procedure codes. Thus, even if an insurer agrees to provide coverage for a new test or treatment in response to a claim appeal, it may take a while until a new procedure code can be established. In the meantime, reimbursement may be provided on the basis of a related procedure code. That may result in a significantly lower payment.

If that occurs, you can ask your doctor and/or the local medical society to work with the insurer to help develop a new procedure code so that payment can be made at the appropriate level. Once the new code has been established, you may need to file a claim appeal to obtain appropriate reimbursement.

DEALING WITH SERIOUS CLAIM PROBLEMS

Following the steps described in this chapter and in previous chapters will help prevent health insurance problems from occurring and will help you solve many of the problems that do occur. However, serious claim problems may nevertheless develop at times.

If a serious health insurance problem occurs and claim appeals to your insurer are unsuccessful, you can contact your county or state medical society, your state Department of Insurance or Department of Health, or an appropriate federal agency. You can also seek help from self-help or advocacy groups, from a private medical claim-processing company, from an attorney, or from your state or federal legislative representatives. (See Chapter 3 for a more detailed discussion of this issue.)

SUMMARY

An insurance policy represents an agreement. In an individual policy, the agreement is between the consumer and the insurance company; in an employer-sponsored group policy, the agreement is between the employer and the insurance company. In either case, the treatments, tests, and services covered by a health insurance policy are always limited and are always subject to detailed policy rules. In order to obtain the health insurance benefits to which you are entitled, you need to understand those policy rules and you need to become familiar with some of the more common claim problems and their possible solutions.

Those problems may include difficulties related to

- yearly deductibles;
- procedure codes;
- the UCR and percentiles;
- secondary insurance benefits;
- claim denials on the grounds that the treatment or service does not represent a covered expense, is not medically necessary, or is experimental.

Fortunately, there are a number of responses that may be effective in such situations. Those responses include the possibility of filing a claim appeal with your insurer, or seeking help from

- your county or state medical society;
- your state Department of Insurance;
- your state Department of Health;
- appropriate federal agencies;
- self-help or advocacy groups;
- a private medical claim-processing company;
- an attorney;
- state or federal legislative representatives.

5

Traditional Individual and Group Plans, Hospital Bills

Years ago, it was fairly easy to deal with hospital (inpatient) claims. When you were admitted to a hospital, all you generally had to do was to give the hospital billing office a copy of your insurance identification card. The hospital then filed the claim with your insurer and took care of all the details. These days, with pre-authorization requirements, co-payments, outpatient pre-admission testing, and other innovations, a consumer has to be closely involved in order to be certain that everything is progressing properly in terms of the billing and claim-filing process.

BECOMING FAMILIAR WITH POLICY RULES

It's essential that you understand your health insurance policy rules in regard to reimbursement for hospital services. For example, you need to determine whether your policy provides coverage for a private hospital room in some circumstances or for a semi-private room only. In addition, you need to determine the extent to which coverage is provided for intensive care, and you need to determine whether or not the policy requires that pre-admission testing be performed prior to hospitalization in a non-emergency situation.

Most importantly, it's essential to determine whether your health insurance policy requires that you, a family member, or a hospital representative call your insurance company prior to admission to a hospital or prior to a transfer to a hospital inten-sive care unit. That requirement is generally referred to as **pre-authorization.** Policies that require pre-authorization may pro-vide for penalties for failing to call prior to hospitalization, in-cluding a significant reduction in benefits. You also need to de-termine what the process is for obtaining such pre-authori-zation, particularly on weekends, holidays, and in emergency situations.

If your policy requires pre-authorization prior to hospital-ization, when you call the insurance company it's essential that you write down the date, the time, and the name of the person with whom you have spoken. That will help to ensure that there will be a record of the telephone call if questions occur later about whether pre-authorization was obtained. Since decisions in regard to hospitalization are often made on an emergency basis, it's important to research these issues well in advance of the need for the information and to place the answers in your information file.

CHECKING THE HOSPITAL BILL

These days, hospitals generally file claims for inpatient services directly with insurance companies, and they often re-ceive payment directly from the insurer. In some ways, that makes it easier for the consumer, since there are no claim forms for consumers to fill out for a hospital bill. However, it also means that a consumer who receives inpatient services needs to take particular care to make certain that the hospital bill is filed correctly, and that it is accurate. For that reason, it's generally helpful to request a copy of your hospital bill, even in situations in which the hospital may take responsibility for filing the claim with your insurer.

Check the hospital bill carefully to make certain that it does not contain any errors. Depending on the policy, a consumer may be responsible for a percentage of the bill, including a percentage of any charges that may have been added by er-ror. Some of the items listed on the bill will be self-explanatory.

Other items may be abbreviated, or may be listed only by code name or number.

Table 12 represents an example of the kind of bill that a hospital might send to an insurance company. It includes only the cost of services, tests, and equipment supplied by the hospital. Doctors' services are billed separately. In this hypothetical case, surgery was involved, and the patient also had other medical problems (See Table 12).

The abbreviation "Med-Surg-Semi-Prvt" in Table 12 refers to the cost of a semi-private room in the hospital's medical-surgical unit. The "6" in the "Comments" section refers to the time period, six days in this case. "Phrmcy" (pharmacy) refers to the cost of medications. "Med Supplies" includes the cost of such items as tape and bandages.

"Med Tests" includes expenses related to laboratory tests conducted during the time the patient was in the hospital. "CT" refers to a CAT scan (computerized axial tomography). "OR" refers to expenses related to the use of the operating room during surgery. "Blood" includes the cost of storing and processing blood that was used in a blood transfusion related to surgery.

"U-S" refers to the use of ultrasound equipment. In this case, the diagnostic tests were directly related to the surgery. "Recvry" refers to expenses related to the use of the recovery room immediately following surgery. "Tel" includes the cost of having a telephone near the patient's bed. Once again, the "6" in the "Comments" section refers to the fact that the telephone was in place for six days. Expenses related to telephone use are not generally covered by health insurance policies.

If the insurer requests an **itemized bill,** a bill such as the one presented in Table 12 would probably be between ten and thirty pages in length. It would include details related to specific medications, medical or surgical supplies, laboratory tests, blood transfusions, and other procedures. Many hospitals use different abbreviations. If a particular item listed on a hospital bill is unclear, ask the hospital billing office for an explanation.

Table 12
A Hypothetical Hospital Bill

Hospital: (Name of hospital)
Insurer: (Name of insurance company)
Insured/Patient: (Name of the policyholder and the patient)
Patient's Insurance Company ID Number: (Identification number)
Procedure Code: (Numerical procedure code)

Description	Cost	Comments
Med-Surg-Semi-Prvt	$6,000	6
Phrmcy	$1,900	
Med Supplies	$4,120	
Med Tests	$3,573	
X-ray	$ 57	
CT	$1,500	
OR	$1,196	
Blood	$ 251	
U-S	$1,620	
Recvry	$1,100	
Tel	$ 120	6

When you review your hospital bill, make certain you understand each of the items listed. If there appears to be an error, notify both the hospital and the insurance company as soon as possible. That notification should be made in writing, not by telephone, so that there is a permanent record of the report. Be certain to keep a copy of your letter.

SECONDARY INSURERS AND HOSPITAL CLAIMS

Although hospitals may take responsibility for filing a claim for hospital services with a consumer's primary insurer, some hospitals do not take responsibility for filing the claim with the consumer's secondary insurer. Thus, if you have secondary insurance coverage—under a spouse's health insurance policy, for example—it's important to check with the hospital billing office to determine whether the hospital will take responsibility for filing your secondary insurance claim. If the hospital billing office does not routinely file such claims, you will have to file the claim with your secondary insurer.

In order to file the claim, you'll need a copy of the hospital bill and a copy of the Explanation of Benefits Statement from your primary insurer. If you don't have a copy of the hospital bill, you can obtain it from the hospital billing office. Since insurers sometimes pay hospitals either electronically or with a single check that's intended to cover claims for all hospital patients during a specific period of time, the hospital billing office will probably not have a copy of your EOBS. If you do not have a copy, you can request one from your primary insurer.

A HOSPITAL STAY MAY PRODUCE A MULTITUDE OF BILLS

Years ago, patients who were not covered by health insurance often received a single bill when they left the hospital. If a patient was covered by health insurance, only a single bill was generally sent to the insurer. That bill included charges for the hospital room, food, medications, nursing care, and the use of hospital facilities, as well as charges for the services of the doctors and surgeons who provided treatment. Hospitals don't always work that way any more. Instead, a hospital may bill the patient only for the cost of the room, food, medication, nursing care, supplies, and the use of hospital facilities. Each of the doctors who provided treatment in the hospital may send a separate bill.

In addition, while the hospital may file the bill for hospital services directly with your insurance company, the insurance information that you gave to the hospital will not necessarily be given to the doctors who provided treatment. Thus, the bills from those doctors may be sent to you, not to your insurer. When you receive the bills, you can either provide each of the doctors' offices with your insurance information so that they can file the claims with your insurer, or you can file the claims on your own.

For example, let's assume that you accidentally trip while stepping off the sidewalk and that you're injured in the fall. You're taken by ambulance to the emergency room of the local hospital, where you are treated for a fractured arm and a possible head injury. You're eventually admitted to the hospital overnight for observation and further tests—including an X-ray of your arm and your head—and you're released the next morning. During your brief hospital stay, treatment would probably have been provided by an emergency room doctor, a radiologist, an orthopedic surgeon, and a neurologist. Each of those doctors may send you a separate bill, in addition to the bill from the hospital. While the hospital may file the claim for hospital services with your insurer, you may be responsible for filing the claim for the emergency room doctor, the radiologist, the orthopedic surgeon, and the neurologist.

PAYING HOSPITAL BILLS

If you're certain that your health insurance will cover a substantial portion of your hospital bill, it's not generally a good idea for you to pay the bill until both your primary and secondary insurance companies have processed the claim. Many hospitals are accustomed to filing claims with insurance companies on a direct basis, and many insurers routinely send payments directly to the hospital. If you pay the hospital bill before your insurer has processed it, you may unintentionally interfere with that system. If both you and your insurer eventually pay the hospital, you may have to go through a complex process to resolve the problem. That can take time, and may involve a great deal of paperwork.

For example, I recently helped a reader of my newspaper column with a problem involving duplicate payments to a hospital. She had been in the hospital for an extended period. She was covered by both a primary and a secondary insurer, and the primary insurer paid most of the bill. However, there was a balance of almost $2,000 remaining.

A few weeks after the hospital stay, the hospital sent her a bill for that balance. Since the hospital did not generally file secondary insurance claims, she paid the $2,000 bill with her personal check, and she filed the claim with her secondary insurer. The secondary insurer provided reimbursement for the full amount of the claim, but sent the check directly to the hospital.

Since the bill had already been paid in full as far as the hospital was concerned, the hospital apparently assumed that the check was a duplicate sent in error and returned it to the insurance company. It took a number of months to resolve the problem. This case represents a good illustration of the need to allow both primary and secondary insurers to fully process hospital claims before paying the remaining balance.

However, until your insurance company pays the bill, you may receive bills or letters from the hospital requesting immediate payment. Those may be computer-generated messages, and should not be taken personally. If your insurer does not pay the bill within a reasonable period of time, you will need to respond to those notices. At that point, you'll need to work with the hospital billing office and the insurer to identify and correct the problem.

If your insurer does not pay the bill quickly, file an immediate claim appeal with the insurance company. It's important to deal with an unpaid hospital bill before the hospital turns the matter over to a collection agency, since that can produce unnecessary complications. If your insurer does not pay the hospital bill—even after you've filed a claim appeal—and you receive a letter from the hospital suggesting that they are planning to turn the bill over to a collection agency, it's essential to respond immediately and to talk with the hospital billing office and with your insurer to try to resolve the problem. (See Chapter 3 for information on resolving claims problems.) If you need additional help, you can consult an appropriate state or federal agency, your county or state medical society, a private claim-processing company, or an attorney.

Once your primary and secondary insurer have fully processed the claim and have provided the appropriate reimbursement for the hospital bill, it's important to pay any remaining balance quickly. In addition to co-payments, that balance may include expenses related to the use of a telephone, the cost of a television rental, and similar expenses that are not usually covered by health insurance policies.

MAINTAINING COPIES OF HOSPITAL BILLS

Once a hospital bill has been paid, it's essential to maintain copies of all records related to the claim, including bills, Explanation of Benefit Statements, operative reports, and letters. Some insurance companies periodically review hospital claims, even though the bill may already have been paid. That review may include claims processed several years earlier. If the insurance company review determines that a claim was incorrectly paid to a hospital, or that the paperwork or documentation is not complete, the insurer may **rescind** the payment—ask the hospital to return the money—without notifying you in advance. Once the payment has been rescinded, the hospital may request that you pay the bill in full.

You may receive the first such request from the hospital two or three years after your hospital admission. At that point, you'll need to talk with your insurer to try to immediately identify the problem, and you may need to file a claim appeal. In order to do that, you'll need the records. If you haven't kept copies of those records, you'll have to try to obtain them from the insurer and the hospital billing office. However, after two or three years, those records may have been transferred to a storage area or placed on microfiche. It could take months to obtain copies.

If you keep copies of all hospital records, in many cases you may be able to resolve such problems quickly. For example, I recently helped a reader resolve a problem that involved a bill related to a hospital stay for an extended period of time more than five years earlier. In that case, the insurer had paid most of the bill. However, there was still a balance of almost $10,000. The insurer continued to deny the claim. Five years later, the hospital sent the reader a notice requesting immediate payment.

As it turned out, the bill was covered by the individual's insurance policy. The claim denial was based only on the insurer's requirements for additional documentation from the hospital. The hospital insisted that they had sent copies of the records to the insurer. However, the insurer claimed that they had received some of the records, but that they needed additional documentation.

Fortunately, the reader had kept copies of all of the records related to the hospital stay. Those records made it possible for a hospital billing department supervisor to locate the official records quickly, and to ensure that the appropriate documentation was forwarded to the insurer.

The question of how long you need to maintain copies of records related to a hospital stay is a difficult one to answer. I have worked with readers of my newspaper column in situations in which insurers rescinded payment for hospital services four or five years after the hospitalization had originally occurred. Certainly, given those experiences, it may be a good idea to keep such records for at least five years.

SUMMARY

Dealing with hospital bills has become far more complex than it once was. Given the current cost of hospital-based care, it's essential that you understand the rules under which your insurance policy operates and the specific coverage provided by your policy for hospital services. Although many claims for such services are reimbursed routinely, there are also a variety of problems that can occur. Those problems may include

- difficulty in obtaining pre-authorization, or in demonstrating that such pre-authorization was obtained;
- possible errors on hospital bills, or in the way such bills have been filed with the insurer;
- obtaining benefits from your secondary insurer;
- knowing when to pay a hospital bill;
- dealing with a situation in which your insurer has rescinded payment for a hospital bill.

In some cases, problems can be prevented by carefully following the rules of your health insurance policy. If problems do occur, possible solutions include filing a claim appeal with your insurer, or seeking help from your county or state medical society, your state Department of Insurance or Department of Health, appropriate federal agencies, self-help or advocacy groups, a private medical claim-processing company, an attorney, or your state or federal legislative representatives.

Given the amount of money involved in claims for a hospital stay, it's important for consumers to pay close attention to the billing and claim-filing process. Consumers who understand the system and who are aware of the potential difficulties can often deal successfully with any problems that may occur.

6
Self-funded Plans

A **self-funded plan** is a benefit plan established by a corporation, a union, an association, or a state or municipal government agency. Such plans play an important role in the American health insurance system. At present, the majority of large employers offer benefits through such plans.

Self-funded plans may differ significantly from each other. For example, some self-funded plans may offer a managed care approach within the self-funded plan framework; others may offer a more traditional approach. Some self-funded plans may be administered directly by the plan sponsor—the corporation, union, association, or state or municipal government agency—while others may be administered by a **plan administrator** such as an insurance company.

Self-funded plans also differ significantly from both traditional health insurance plans and managed care plans in a number of ways. First, traditional health insurance plans or managed care plans are generally designed by an insurer, and the insurer makes benefit-related decisions in terms of the plan rules. However, a self-funded plan is usually designed by the plan sponsor, a corporation, a union, an association, or a state or municipal government agency. If an insurance company serves as the plan administrator for a self-funded plan, the company generally acts only as the administrator, not as the insurer. In that capacity, the insurance company carries out the plan rules established by the sponsor.

Second, self-funded plans are regulated under **ERISA** (the federal **Employee Retirement Income Security Act**) in terms of benefit-related issues, and are generally exempt from state laws and regulations related to benefits. In many cases, self-funded plans appear to offer benefits that are equal to—or more comprehensive than—traditional health insurance policies or managed care plans. However, the exemption from state laws and regulations in relation to benefits makes it important to carefully review the plan provisions to ensure that you understand the benefits and limitations.

The fact that self-funded plans are regulated under federal law in terms of benefit-related issues also affects the appeals process. For example, in the case of a decision made by a traditional insurer or a managed care plan dealing with claims or benefits, the first step in the appeals process is to file an appeal with the insurer or the managed care plan itself. Once those appeals have been exhausted, further appeals can be filed with the state Department of Insurance or the state Department of Health, or with other organizations.

However, in the case of a decision made by a self-funded plan, the first step in the appeals process is to file an appeal with the plan administrator or the plan sponsor. Once appeals to the plan administrator and plan sponsor have been exhausted, further appeals should be filed with the Pension and Welfare Benefits Administration of the United States Department of Labor (See Appendix B). If those appeals are unsuccessful, the next step may be to consult an attorney.

Third, the money used to pay claims in a self-funded plan generally comes from the plan sponsor—the corporation, union, association, or government agency—rather than from an insurance company. In order to cover unexpectedly high medical claims, some self-funded plans may make use of **reinsurance programs.** Reinsurance provides coverage for claims above a pre-set amount. (See Table 13 for a comparison of self-funded plans and traditional health insurance plans.)

Table 13
Comparison of Self-funded Plans and Traditional Health Insurance Plans

Traditional Plan	Self-funded Plan
Established by an insurance company	Established by a plan sponsor such as a corporation, a union, an association, or a state or municipal government agency
Regulated by state agencies, including the state Department of Insurance, the state Department of Health, or by special state health insurance boards	Regulated through ERISA (the federal Employee Retirement Income Security Act), implemented by the Pension and Welfare Benefits Administration of the U.S. Department of Labor
Claims paid by the insurance company	Claims paid by the plan sponsor (the sponsor may also have a reinsurance program)
Appeals may be filed with the insurer, the state Department of Insurance, the state Department of Health, or with other organizations	Appeals may be filed with the plan administrator, the plan sponsor, or the Pension and Welfare Benefits Administration of the United States Department of Labor

The Portability and Accountability Act, passed in 1996, provides a series of new protections for consumers who are covered by self-funded plans. For example, the act generally requires self-funded plans to notify participants of any significant reduction in benefits within sixty days or to issue a regular plan description every ninety days. The act also generally prohibits self-funded plans and insurance companies from refusing to renew coverage for an individual on the basis of a disability. In addition, both self-funded plans and insurance companies are generally prohibited from imposing rules that discriminate against an individual on the basis of a disability.

In some cases, the Americans with Disabilities Act may also affect the decisions that self-funded plans can make in terms of benefits for an individual with a disability. However, those laws do not appear to prohibit self-funded plans or insurance companies from limiting specific benefits, as long as the limitations apply to all people insured under the plan rather than to a specific individual.

Since self-funded plans are not regulated by state laws or regulations in terms of benefits, they appear to present a unique situation for consumers. However, corporations, unions, associations, and government agencies are not generally required to offer health benefits. Since self-funded plans appear to offer significantly reduced administrative and other costs, they may allow a plan sponsor to offer health benefits in a situation in which the sponsor might otherwise be unable to provide any coverage at all.

SUMMARY

Self-funded plans represent an important part of the health insurance system in America. In many cases, such plans appear to offer benefits that are equal to—or more comprehensive than—traditional insurance policies or managed care plans. Self-funded plans may also allow for benefits to be offered in situations in which they might not otherwise be available.

However, self-funded plans may present a unique situation for consumers in some ways, since such plans are established by a plan sponsor such as a corporation, a union, an association, or a state or municipal government agency rather than by an insurance company. In addition, self-funded plans are regulated under a federal law called ERISA—the Employee

Retirement Income Security Act—in terms of benefit-related issues, rather than under state law. ERISA is implemented by the Pension and Welfare Benefits Administration of the United States Department of Labor, not by state Departments of Insurance or state Departments of Health. Over the past few years, there have been some important changes in the laws that relate to self-funded plans, particularly in terms of providing additional protections for consumers.

7

Managed Care Plans

The introduction of managed care plans—sometimes referred to as **MCOs (Managed Care Organizations)**—has resulted in enormous changes in the American system of health care.

Originally, **managed care** referred almost exclusively to **HMOs (Health Maintenance Organizations).** However, over the past decade the concept has expanded significantly. In additon to HMOs, the term "managed care" is now often used to refer to any health plan that has a network of doctors, hospitals, and testing centers, and provisions such as a requirement for pre-authorization prior to specific treatments, tests, or services.

At this point, in addition to standard HMOs, managed care plans also include

- HMOs with a Point-of-Service (POS) Option;
- Medicare HMOs;
- Medicaid HMOs;
- Preferred Provider Organizations (PPOs).

Managed care also includes a number of plans that combine various approaches. These days, the term managed care is sometimes used to refer, as well, to those aspects of traditional health insurance policies that have incorporated selected managed care provisions. Such provisions may include requirements for pre-authorization prior to hospital admission, expensive tests, physical therapy, or psychiatric treatment. Some more traditional health insurance plans may also have a provider network. Although consumers who are enrolled in such plans can use non-network providers whenever they wish, consulting providers who are part of the plan network may offer additional cost savings.

At present, approximately 70% of all employees in America who work for medium or large companies are participants in managed care programs of some type. As private managed care plans expand, as the number of Medicare HMOs increases, and as states require a larger percentage of Medicaid recipients to join Medicaid HMOs, managed care is likely to play an increasingly important role in the American health insurance system.

HEALTH MAINTENANCE ORGANIZATIONS (HMOs)

A Health Maintenance Organization may provide medical services in one central building, or such services may be provided through a network of individual doctors, hospitals, and testing centers, with offices scattered over a large geographic area. However, regardless of the particular structure, all of the providers in an HMO generally follow the same network rules.

HMOs may offer some significant advantages to consumers. First, in many cases HMOs may be less expensive than traditional health plans. Second, since there are usually no deductibles for HMO participants, out-of-pocket costs may be far lower. Third, HMO participants are not generally required to file claim forms or to wait for reimbursement. Fourth, since all providers in an HMO network generally follow the same network rules, there is usually no need to be concerned about the possibility that a provider's charge will be considered to be above the UCR (Usual and Customary Rate). Fifth, HMOs often provide coverage for preventive services, including vaccinations, annual physicals, and routine screening tests (See Table 14).

However, in order to obtain full benefits, HMO participants are generally expected to make use of network providers. Participants may also be required to pay a small fee for each visit to a doctor. In addition, coverage for a consultation with a specialist or for medical tests may be available only with the agreement of the **primary care physician.**

The primary care physician is often referred to as the **gatekeeper,** since that physician controls access to medical specialists and to other medical services. In practical terms, that means that in order to consult a neurologist, a psychiatrist, an orthopedic surgeon, a rheumatologist, or other specialist, or in order to arrange for a CAT scan (computerized axial tomography), an MRI (magnetic resonance imaging), or another type of expensive medical test, a patient must generally first obtain the approval of the primary care physician.

If an HMO has a POS (Point-of-Service) Option, participants may be able to occasionally consult out-of-network providers and still receive partial reimbursement. Check with your HMO to determine the specific rules for coverage under the POS option. If a POS option is not available through a particular HMO, patients can always go outside the system to arrange for medical tests or to obtain treatment for a disease or condition. However, they must generally do so at their own expense, unless the HMO grants approval to consult a provider who is not part of the plan network.

Table 14
Comparison of Traditional Plans and Health Maintenance Organizations

Traditional Plan	HMO
Preventive services are not generally covered	A wide range of preventive services are generally covered, including vaccinations, screening tests, and yearly physicals

Table 14 (Continued)

Traditional Plan	HMO
Out-of-pocket costs may be significantly higher for consumers	Out-of-pocket costs may be significantly lower for consumers
Consumers must file a claim form after each visit to a provider and after each test or service	Claim forms are not usually required as long as network providers are involved
There are often concerns about the possibility that a provider's charge may exceed the insurance company's determination of the UCR	Since network providers follow network rules, consumers need not generally be concerned about issues related to the UCR
There is no need to obtain advance approval prior to consulting a specialist or arranging expensive medical tests, although some traditional plans may require pre-authorization prior to hospitalization	Prior approval by the primary care physician is generally required before consulting a specialist or arranging for expensive medical tests

Under certain circumstances, HMOs may grant approval for a participant to consult an out-of-network provider, particularly if the provider has specialized skills or expertise that are not available within the plan network. However, the process of obtaining such permission may sometimes be difficult and time-consuming.

There are several ongoing controversies in regard to HMOs. One important controversy revolves around the question of whether HMOs are likely to be able to control the costs of medical care in the long run. According to supporters of the HMO concept, the gatekeeper system may eliminate unnecessary tests and services, and the emphasis on preventive care may result in a reduction in the need for hospitalization and expensive treatments. Those aspects of the HMO system may eventually reduce costs considerably. However, not everyone is convinced that HMOs will be able to control the costs of medical care on a long-term basis.

Another major controversy revolves around the question of whether HMOs can offer patients as effective a system of medical care as traditional plans, particularly for people with disabilities or special health care needs. For example, some people have expressed concerns about the degree to which HMOs are likely to be prepared to offer the kinds of services needed by patients with disabilities or conditions such as MS (multiple sclerosis), Down syndrome, autism, post-polio syndrome, or unusual types of heart conditions. In many cases, patients with such illnesses or conditions may require treatment by highly trained specialists, and they may also require a wide range of services. Of course, concerns have been raised, as well, about the degree to which such needs are generally met for patients enrolled in traditional health insurance plans.

Questions have also been raised about the degree to which HMOs are prepared to offer effective treatment for patients with serious mental and emotional illnesses. Those concerns have focused on such issues as requirements for pre-authorization prior to outpatient treatment, limitations on the number of outpatient sessions that may be allowed without additional authorization, and the process of obtaining approval for admission to a psychiatric hospital in an emergency situation.

It's difficult to evaluate these issues, since the rules under which Health Maintenance Organizations operate may differ significantly from one plan to another. Eventually, information on the effectiveness and the economic benefits of HMOs may become available through research. That research may focus on the number of illnesses and conditions experienced by participants in HMOs as compared to patients in traditional plans, the degree to which individuals with serious mental or emotional illnesses require hospitalization, and the long-term costs of medical care in each type of plan. However, it may be a number of years before definitive answers to these questions are available.

In the meantime, organizations such as the **National Committee for Quality Assurance (NCQA)**—an independent, not-for-profit organization—have developed a series of criteria for the accreditation of HMOs. The NCQA is currently in the process of conducting reviews of existing HMO programs. The eventual goal is to provide consumers with additional information so that they can make educated decisions concerning HMOs.

The NCQA has already reviewed more than half of the HMOs in the United States. Such reviews focus on six different areas during the accreditation process, including quality improvement, physician credentials, members rights and responsibilities, preventive health services, utilization management, and medical records.

The NCQA also offers a **"Health Plan Employer Data and Information Set" (HEDIS)** that may prove helpful to consumers who are seeking information about HMOs. HEDIS is a series of standards for measuring the performance of particular managed care plans. Information on HEDIS or on accreditation for specific HMOs is available through the NCQA's Internet site or by calling the NCQA (See Appendix B).

In addition, the federal government has surveyed federal employees in terms of their satisfaction with various HMOs. That information is available to consumers and can be quite helpful, as well (See Appendix B).

However, the available information is not yet complete. Thus, at this point, you'll also have to rely on your own research to evaluate the degree to which a particular HMO may meet your needs. Before joining an HMO, it may be helpful to compare various programs and to discuss plan rules with program representatives. It may also be helpful to try to speak with HMO participants who have health conditions similar to your own to determine their level of satisfaction with the medical care they have received.

It's important, as well, to make certain that there are network providers available in your geographic area—including the types of specialists that you are likely to require—before joining an HMO, and to make certain that the doctor you're considering choosing as your primary care physician has openings for new patients. In addition, it's important to be certain that the hospitals that are part of the HMO network are conveniently located.

PREFERRED PROVIDER ORGANIZATIONS

PPOs (Preferred Provider Organizations) have established provider networks. Consumers must generally make use of the providers in the network in order to allow for maximum reimbursement. However, Preferred Provider Organization rules also permit consumers to see doctors outside the plan network. In such cases, though, a consumer's out-of-pocket costs are likely to be higher than they would be if the consumer consulted a provider who was part of the plan network.

A Preferred Provider Organization may thus provide some of the advantages of a managed care plan when the consumer makes use of network physicians, but it may also offer some of the advantages of a traditional plan by allowing for some cost savings when services are provided by physicians outside the plan network.

DEALING WITH PROBLEMS IN MANAGED CARE

Services and treatments offered through managed care plans are generally handled routinely, with few difficulties. Unfortunately, when participants in managed care plans do experience problems, they may be very difficult to resolve. The problems commonly reported with managed care plans at this point include difficulty in obtaining reimbursement for

- treatment in a hospital emergency room;
- a consultation with a specialist outside of the plan network;
- treatment beyond what the managed care plan may determine to be medically necessary;
- hospitalization or services such as physical therapy—which generally require pre-authorization—in cases in which no pre-authorization was granted.

It's often possible to prevent such problems from occurring by carefully following the rules of the managed care plan, and by keeping careful records of all communications with plan representatives that relate to coverage or reimbursement. If a problem occurs in terms of coverage or reimbursement, it's important to make full use of the managed care plan's appeals system. File a claim appeal at each stage of the process until the issue is resolved, and keep copies of the appeals and the responses you receive. If your appeals are unsuccessful, you may wish to consider the possibility of writing to a supervisor or an executive at the managed care plan.

Supervisors and executives are generally quite knowledgeable about program rules. My experience is that they are often very responsive to consumer problems, as well. In several cases where I've tried to help readers of my newspaper column deal with problems involving managed care plans, I've found that even complex problems were often easily solved once a supervisor or an executive became involved.

If you write to a supervisor or an executive at a managed care plan, make certain that you include all of the relevant information and documentation. Make certain, as well, that your letter stays focused on the issue at hand. A letter that attempts to review all the difficulties you have ever experienced with the managed care plan or with health insurance in general is unlikely to lead to a quick solution of the immediate problem.

Your letter to a supervisor or executive might begin by listing your name, address, phone number, and identification number, and then noting the date of service, the type of treatment or test involved, and a brief description of the problem.

You might then explain why you think the plan's decision was incorrect. Cite specific sections of the policy or other evidence that supports your point of view.

If a supervisor or executive responds with a letter or a telephone call, it's important to remain calm and polite at each stage of the process and to explain the problem as simply and as clearly as possible. If you're feeling angry or upset about the way your claim has been handled, wait until you're feeling calmer before discussing the issue.

If your letter does not resolve the problem, the next step is to write to your state Department of Insurance or Department of Health and ask for their help. Although the structure differs from state to state, one or both of those state agencies are generally responsible for implementing state health insurance laws and regulations that deal with managed care plans in a particular state. If that does not result in a resolution of the problem, you can also write to the American Association of Health Plans (AAHP)—a national organization that represents Health Maintenance Organizations and other types of managed care plans—or to the National Committee for Quality Assurance (NCQA), the organization involved in reviewing HMOs for possible accreditation (See Appendix B). Both the American Association of Health Plans and the National Committee for Quality Assurance have programs that are designed to help consumers solve problems related to HMOs or to other managed care organizations.

There are other organizations and agencies that may be able to offer help and advice, as well, particularly if the problem relates to a child with a disability (See Appendix B). In addition, you can also discuss the problem with an attorney.

SUMMARY

Over the past decade, the movement toward managed care has revolutionized health insurance in America. At this point, many people seem convinced that managed care programs will save significant amounts of money in the long run while continuing to provide excellent health care. Thus, such programs are likely to expand in the future, both in terms of employer-sponsored health insurance plans and government-sponsored plans such as Medicare, Medicaid, and CHAMPUS. As research on the effectiveness and the economics of managed care plans is completed, definitive answers should be available to questions about the managed care approach.

8

CHAMPUS and Medical Savings Accounts

A variety of specialized programs have been established to meet health insurance needs in specific situations. For example, the federal government has developed a special health benefit program for families of armed forces personnel and for retired members of the armed forces. In addition, Medical Savings Accounts and high-deductible health insurance plans have recently been developed to provide a new approach to health insurance that includes the possibility of special tax benefits to individual participants.

CHAMPUS

CHAMPUS, the **Civilian Health and Medical Program of the Uniformed Services,** is a health benefit program established by the federal government for families of armed forces personnel and for retired members of the armed forces.

At present, there are two CHAMPUS systems in operation. There's an older, traditional system—now generally referred to either as CHAMPUS or as **Tri-Care Standard**—and a new managed care system called **Tri-Care Prime.** The traditional system currently operates primarily in the northeast, while Tri-Care Prime operates in most other areas of the country.

In many ways, the traditional CHAMPUS system seems to follow the basic structure of the Medicare program (See Chapter 9). Individuals choose their own providers, and claims are processed by local plan administrators rather than by a single national processing center. Furthermore, CHAMPUS categorizes providers as either participating providers or nonparticipating providers, just as Medicare does.

Participating providers accept the CHAMPUS allowable amount, the amount that CHAMPUS has determined to be appropriate for a particular treatment or service. The individual is generally responsible for the deductible and the co-payment. Nonparticipating providers are permitted to charge up to 115% of the CHAMPUS allowable amount (15% above the allowable amount). In addition, both participating providers and nonparticipating providers generally file claims directly with local CHAMPUS plan administrators. That helps to reduce the burden for the consumer in regard to claim-filing, although it's still essential for individuals to keep accurate records of all medical bills and claims.

Participants in the traditional program also have a PPO (Preferred Provider Organization) option called **Tri-Care Extra.** The PPO option allows participants to consult a provider within the PPO network when they wish. Consulting a network provider may result in significant cost-savings. PPO participants can consult out-of-network providers, as well.

Tri-Care Prime centers are already in operation in two-thirds of the country, particularly in the south, southeast, and west. Additional Tri-Care Prime centers are scheduled to be established in the remaining areas of the country within the next few years. Eventually, Tri-Care Prime is expected to become one of the standard ways of providing medical care to eligible individuals throughout the country.

As with most managed care plans, the Tri-Care Prime system offers important benefits to participants. For example, there are usually no claim forms to fill out, and some preventive care—screening tests, for example—is usually covered. However, Tri-Care participants must generally obtain approval from their primary care physician for tests and consultations with a specialist.

CHAMPUS does not operate Tri-Care centers directly. Instead, CHAMPUS contracts with various agencies and organizations to administer Tri-Care in different areas of the country.

The basic rules of the CHAMPUS program are described in the *CHAMPUS Handbook*. If you live near a military base, you may be able to obtain a copy of that handbook from the base health benefits advisor. You can also order the book directly from the national Tri-Care Support office (See Appendix B).

The CHAMPUS programs reportedly work reasonably well for most routine claims. However, as with any program, there are times when errors, misunderstandings, or disagreements may occur. If you're having difficulty obtaining reimbursement or medical services that you think are appropriate under the CHAMPUS system, there is an established appeals procedure.

The first step is to file a claim appeal with the company that originally processed the claim. If services were provided through the traditional CHAMPUS program, the claim appeal should be filed with the local plan administrator. If services were provided through the newer program, the claim appeal should be filed with the local Tri-Care center. If those claim appeals are unsuccessful, you can file a claim appeal directly with the national Tri-Care Support office (See Appendix B).

When filing a claim appeal, it's essential to include copies of all EOBS (Explanation of Benefits Statements) and medical bills, as well as a brief explanation of the problem. While the appeals are being processed, it's important to continue to keep detailed records of all medical bills, even when the claims are filed by the providers. If you have specific questions about CHAMPUS rules, you can call the national Tri-Care Support office for further information (See Appendix B).

MEDICAL SAVINGS ACCOUNTS

Medical Savings Accounts (MSAs), established as part of the Portability and Accountability Act, represent a new concept in the American system of health insurance. As of January 1,

1997, the act allows eligible individuals to participate in special **high-deductible health insurance plans** and to deposit funds in special Medical Savings Accounts. Under the act, funds deposited in an MSA may receive special treatment in terms of federal income taxes.

The federal government designed MSAs as a pilot project, covering only a four-year period (from January 1, 1997 to December 31, 2000). The program is limited to a maximum of 750,000 participants. There are a variety of specialized rules that apply if the number of participants exceeds that maximum.

During the time the pilot project is in operation, the United States Department of the Treasury and the General Accounting Office are expected to evaluate the effects of Medical Savings Accounts on federal revenues, on individuals, and on families. At the end of the pilot project, Congress will have an opportunity to review the reports of those agencies and to decide if the Medical Savings Account program should continue.

At that point, Congress may decide to continue the Medical Savings Account program as it currently exists for another few years. Congress may decide, as well, to expand or decrease the number of potential participants who are allowed to purchase high-deductible health insurance policies and to establish Medical Savings Accounts, or to modify the rules that relate to MSAs. Congress may also decide to eliminate the MSA approach completely or to make the combination of Medical Savings Accounts and high-deductible health insurance policies a permanent part of the American system of health insurance.

If you're considering the possibility of participating in the Medical Savings Account program, the complexity of the current tax laws makes it essential that you review your situation with an accountant and an attorney before making a decision. Since the program is limited in terms of the number of MSA accounts that will be permitted, it's important to begin that review as soon as possible.

Part III

MEDICARE AND MEDICARE-RELATED PROGRAMS

9

Medicare

Medicare is one of the major components of the American system of health insurance. It provides health insurance coverage for senior citizens, for some people who are no longer able to work due to disability, and for some children and adults with End-Stage Renal Disease (ESRD) who require kidney dialysis treatments.

Certain aspects of the Medicare system are now standardized. For example, medical providers generally file claims directly with Medicare, and payments are usually sent directly to providers. After Medicare has processed a claim, the Medicare beneficiary generally receives an **EOMBS (Explanation of Medicare Benefits Statement)** from Medicare.

If a Medicare beneficiary has a Medigap policy or a secondary health insurance policy that acts as a Medicare supplement—for example, an employer-sponsored group health insurance plan that continues after an individual retires—Medicare may automatically forward the claim to that insurer in certain cases, as long as the individual's identification number and insurance company information are listed on the Medicare claim form. (See Chapter 10 for a detailed discussion of Medigap policies and secondary health insurance policies.) The Medicare beneficiary will then receive an EOBS (Explanation of Benefits Statement) from the Medigap or secondary insurer, and a bill from the medical provider for any remaining balance.

Medicare has established a series of rules that apply to outpatient claims related to doctors' office visits and medical tests. For example, Medicare lists an **allowable amount** for each service, test, or procedure. The specific rules that apply to that allowable amount depend on whether the medical provider—the doctor or testing center—is a **participating provider** or a **nonparticipating provider.**

A participating provider accepts the Medicare allowable amount as the fee. In that case, the provider is said to accept assignment. The Medicare beneficiary generally pays only the deductible—if it has not yet been met for the year—and the co-insurance. Medicare pays the balance. The allowable amount is generally listed on the EOMBS.

A nonparticipating provider does not accept the Medicare allowable amount as the total fee. In that situation, the provider does not accept assignment. A nonparticipating provider is allowed to charge a Medicare beneficiary a maximum of an additional 15% above the Medicare allowable amount (115% of that amount), in addition to the usual deductible and co-insurance amounts.

That 115% rule is known as the **limiting charge.** The additional 15% above the Medicare allowable amount is referred to as the **excess charge.** A simple way to make sense of the limiting charge is to view it in terms of dollars rather than in terms of percentages. From that point of view, the limiting charge permits a provider to charge a maximum of an additional $15—the excess charge—for each $100 of the Medicare allowable amount.

For example, let's assume that the Medicare allowable amount for a specific treatment provided by a doctor is $200. Once the beneficiary's yearly deductible has been met, a doctor who accepts assignment—a participating provider—can generally bill the Medicare beneficiary only for the co-insurance, regardless of the standard fee that might be charged to a patient who was not covered by Medicare. However, if the doctor does not accept assignment—a nonparticipating provider—he can charge the patient for the co-insurance plus an additional $30 (15% of the allowable amount of $200).

Although the Medicare system works quite well in the majority of cases, at times it can be complex and confusing. In addition, communication between Medicare and Medicare beneficiaries sometimes leaves a great deal to be desired. As a result, it can sometimes be difficult to solve problems that do occur.

The complexity and the communications difficulties seem to result from a number of factors. To begin with, the Medicare system is inherently complicated in terms of its basic design. For example, instead of being developed as a single integrated program, Medicare is composed of two separate programs. **Medicare: Part A** focuses on providing coverage for hospital-based (inpatient) treatment. **Medicare: Part B** focuses on providing coverage for outpatient treatment, including doctors' visits and medical tests. Each program follows different rules and has different deductibles and co-insurance amounts.

In addition, the Medicare claim-processing system is administered by a series of local plan administrators rather than by a singe national agency. In some cases, those administrators may have decision-making authority on certain issues. For example, although the federal **Health Care Financing Administration** (**HCFA**)—the federal agency that regulates Medicare—sets national policy in terms of coverage for many tests and procedures, in some cases decisions related to coverage for new tests for which HCFA has not yet issued policies may be left to local Medicare plan administrators. As a result, while reimbursement for certain medical tests may be available to Medicare beneficiaries in one part of the country, reimbursement for similar tests may not be available to beneficiaries in other parts of the country.

Although most Medicare: Part B claims are generally processed through a specific local plan administrator, claims for durable medical equipment—manual and power wheelchairs, crutches, hospital beds, and other equipment—are usually processed through a completely separate Medicare regional administrator.

Such claims may be subject to different rules and procedures, both in comparison with other Medicare claims and with similar claims processed under private insurance policies. For example, Medicare's definition of medical necessity may differ from the definition used in many private insurance policies.

In general, to qualify for Medicare coverage for medical equipment, the equipment must be needed for use within the home. Thus, an individual with severe arthritis who can walk short distances but who may need a power wheelchair for longer distances outside of the house might not qualify for coverage for the wheelchair under Medicare's definition of medical necessity. However, an individual with the same disability might meet the definition of medical necessity used by many private insurance policies. Thus, although the power wheelchair might not be covered by Medicare, it might be covered by such policies. (See Chapter 10 for a discussion of how the application of Medicare's definition of medical necessity for a power wheelchair might affect coverage under a Medigap policy or under an employer-sponsored group health insurance policy that continues after retirement and that acts as a Medicare supplement.)

Medicare may also pay for certain types of home health care, including skilled nursing services, administration of medication, management of a health care plan for a patient, and a variety of other services. To qualify for home health care you must be able to meet a number of qualifications. You must also be confined to your house. However, in terms of Medicare's definition, in some cases being confined to your house may simply mean that you are unable to leave your house without help from another person and without using a wheelchair or other assistive device, but that you do occasionally leave your house for essential appointments. (Check with Medicare to determine the rules for a specific situation.)

The enormous number of complex rules and regulations in the Medicare system creates a great deal of confusion for Medicare beneficiaries. When you finally think you've begun to understand the rules, you find that many of them have exceptions or have been changed.

For example, there are exceptions to the limiting charge rule. Ordinarily, a provider who does not accept assignment cannot charge a Medicare beneficiary more than 115% of the Medicare allowable amount. However, under current Medicare regulations, when occupational therapy is provided by an independent occupational therapist, the limiting charge may apply only to the first $900, the maximum amount that Medicare will generally consider for payment each year for such therapy. Bills above that $900 amount during the same year can reflect the occupational therapist's standard fee. In such situations, the Medicare limiting charge rule does not apply.

There are exceptions to the general rules that govern the Medicare claim-processing system, as well, particularly in terms of Explanation of Benefits Statements. For example, Medicare rules generally provide for full payment to laboratories for many standard tests. For that reason, Medicare may pay laboratories directly. However, in many cases Medicare beneficiaries report that they do not receive an EOMBS for claims for laboratory tests unless they specifically request one from Medicare.

In addition, there is an enormous amount of confusion concerning the question of whether Medicare represents a beneficiary's primary or secondary insurer in situations in which the beneficiary's spouse is covered by an employer-sponsored group health insurance plan. Eliminating that confusion would help many Medicare beneficiaries make sense of the claim-processing system, and might help save a great deal of money.

Under current rules, if the spouse of a Medicare beneficiary is working, and is covered by an employer-sponsored group health insurance plan, the question of whether Medicare is primary or secondary for the Medicare beneficiary depends on three factors: The number of employees in the spouse's company, the age of the Medicare beneficiary, and whether the beneficiary is covered by Medicare as a result of retirement or as a result of a disability.

If a Medicare beneficiary is over age 65, and the beneficiary's spouse is employed and is covered by an employer-sponsored group health insurance policy, Medicare generally becomes the beneficiary's secondary insurer whenever the spouse's company has more than 20 full-time employees. In that case, the spouse's employer-sponsored group health insurance policy represents the Medicare beneficiary's primary insurer. However, if the spouse's company has less than 20 full-time employees, Medicare generally represents the beneficiary's primary insurer.

If the individual is under 65 and is covered by Medicare as a result of a disability, Medicare represents the beneficiary's secondary insurer if the spouse's company has more than 100 full-time employees. In that case, the spouse's employer-sponsored group health insurance plan represents the beneficiary's primary insurer. However, if the spouse's company has less than 100 full-time employees, Medicare represents the beneficiary's primary insurer.

There are also a variety of exceptions to those rules, as there are with many Medicare rules. For example, if the disability involves ESRD (End-Stage Renal Disease), an entirely different set of rules apply. In addition, Medicare may become the secondary insurer in many cases if a Medicare beneficiary has a disability and is also covered for treatments, services, or medical equipment under workman's compensation, liability insurance, veterans' benefits, or other insurance coverage. To make things even more confusing, all of those rules are subject to change. In fact, there have been recent discussions on the federal level of the possibility of revising the rules that relate to the question of when Medicare becomes the secondary insurer in certain cases.

An enormous amount of chaos results from the complex nature of these rules, particularly for Medicare beneficiaries whose spouses work on a full-time basis and who try desperately to figure out if Medicare is their primary or secondary insurer. As a result of the confusion, Medicare beneficiaries may file their medical claims in the wrong order, with claims going to the secondary insurer before the primary insurer has processed them. It can take months to straighten out the resulting problems. In addition to the frustration that the system causes for beneficiaries, it may also cost both private health insurers and Medicare a great deal of money, as insurance company and Medicare personnel process and re-process the bills.

Clearly, the rules could be simplified without much difficulty. In the meantime, if you are uncertain whether Medicare or another insurance company represents your primary insurer, call or write to Medicare or to an organization such as the **Medicare Rights Center** or the **United Seniors Health Cooperative.** You can also get in touch with the state-sponsored health insurance counseling service for Medicare beneficiaries in your area (See Appendix B).

The rules regarding coverage of claims for medical care outside of the United States are also complex. The general rule is that Medicare does not provide coverage for medical care outside of the United States. However, there are several exceptions to that rule. For example, Medicare may provide coverage for emergency medical care received in a Canadian or Mexican hospital if a Medicare beneficiary lives near the Canadian or Mexican border, and if the Canadian or Mexican hospital is closer than the nearest hospital in the United States.

Let's assume that a Medicare beneficiary lives in upstate New York, near the Canadian border, that there's a Canadian hospital just across the border, and that the nearest American hospital is twenty or thirty miles away. If the individual has a serious accident or experiences severe chest pains—the beginning of a heart attack—in the middle of the night and decides to go to the Canadian hospital for treatment because it's closer, Medicare may provide reimbursement.

The same provision applies to Medicare beneficiaries who live in Texas, near the Mexican border. As long as the Canadian or Mexican hospital is significantly closer than the nearest American hospital, and as long as the Medicare beneficiary is being treated for a medical emergency, Medicare may consider providing coverage. Decisions are made on a case-by-case basis.

Medicare may also provide coverage for emergency medical care received at a Canadian hospital for a Medicare beneficiary who is in the process of traveling through Canada on the way to or from Alaska. However, that provision applies only if the individual is traveling by a direct route to or from Alaska, and if the Canadian hospital is closer than the nearest hospital in the United States.

At this point, the Medicare system is so complicated that it can take months to straighten out errors. For example, Medicare may receive information about beneficiaries from a variety of sources, including other government agencies. In some cases, that information may be incorrect or outdated. However, once the information gets into the system, it can be very difficult to have it corrected. In the meantime, claims are often denied on the basis of the erroneous information.

As a result, even widows or widowers who are retired and who have been covered by Medicare for years may find that their claims are suddenly rejected. In some cases, Medicare may insist that it does not represent the individual's primary carrier because the person's spouse—who may, in fact, have died many years before—is covered by an employer-sponsored group health insurance program, or because the individual is working on a full-time basis, or is no longer eligible for Medicare benefits.

Unfortunately, writing to Medicare and explaining the actual situation does not always seem to lead to a successful resolution of the problem. Although it would be simple for Medicare to establish a single national toll-free number for beneficiaries to call in order to quickly correct errors of this type, such a system has not yet been established.

Developing a more efficient system for dealing with fraud, billing errors, and overpayments would also save a significant amount of money. Over the years, Medicare has instituted a variety of mechanisms to prevent and deal with such problems.

However, although those mechanisms have been effective in some cases, there also appear to be a number of circumstances in which they don't seem to work very well.

The Portability and Accountability Act, passed in the summer of 1996, attempts to deal with the problem of fraud by providing for the establishment of a new **Medicare fraud prevention program** and a new **Medicare Beneficiary Incentive Program.**

The fraud prevention program is designed to investigate fraud and payment errors. For the most part, the program is likely to affect providers rather than beneficiaries, although there may be a new educational program for beneficiaries, as well. That program is designed to help increase beneficiaries' understanding of Medicare rules.

The Medicare Beneficiary Incentive Program affects beneficiaries directly. The program is designed to encourage Medicare beneficiaries to report possible cases of fraud. The basic concept is that if those reports result in a recovery of funds, the Medicare beneficiary who originally made the report may receive a portion of those funds. Until that program is fully developed, Medicare beneficiaries can continue to report cases of possible fraud to the Medicare Inspector-General (See Appendix B).

The Medicare Beneficiary Incentive Program is also intended to encourage Medicare beneficiaries to recommend changes in program rules that may save money. The Portability and Accountability Act provided that Medicare may also share a portion of those savings with the beneficiary who originally suggested the idea.

While the government has been willing to begin dealing with the issue of Medicare finances, it seems reluctant to deal with the administrative difficulties that have resulted from the existing system of rules, regulations, and exceptions. In the meantime, the complex structure of the Medicare program continues to create confusion and makes the system far more difficult for consumers than it needs to be.

Fortunately, there is help available for Medicare beneficiaries who are experiencing difficulties. The Medicare appeals system is designed to help consumers deal with situations in which an error has occurred, or in which a claim has not been processed properly. The first step in that system is to file a claim appeal with the local carrier that processed the claim. If that's unsuccessful, a Medicare decision can be appealed further by requesting a **Fair Hearing** or by filing an appeal with an **Administrative Law Judge** or with the **Appeals Council.** However, in many cases, that appeals system can be complicated and time-consuming.

Organizations such as the Medicare Rights Center and the United Seniors Health Cooperative can also help by providing information and advice in dealing with Medicare problems (See Appendix B). These organizations can also offer up-to-date information on specific Medicare rules and programs.

In addition, each state has a free health insurance counseling service designed to provide help and advice to Medicare beneficiaries. The program offers help through trained volunteers. The program is referred to by a different official name in each state, but is generally coordinated by the state Department of Insurance, the Division on Aging, the Division of Senior Services, or the Department of Human Services. Check with those agencies in your state for further information on the state's counseling program for Medicare beneficiaries. The *Medicare Handbook*, available at your local Social Security office, includes a list of the telephone numbers of agencies that coordinate the Medicare health insurance counseling program in each state.

During August of 1997, the federal government made a series of changes in the Medicare program, including the possible development of Medical Savings Accounts, provider-sponsored organizations, and other new types of plans. In addition, the government was in the process of considering the possibility of extending the open-enrollment period during which Medicare beneficiaries can choose a Medigap plan. Check with your state-sponsored counseling service, with the Medicare Rights Center, or with the United Seniors Health

Cooperative for up-to-date information on these issues.

SUMMARY

Certain aspects of the traditional Medicare system have now become standardized, including the process of billing and reimbursement. However, the overall Medicare program has become so complex that it often creates a great deal of unnecessary difficulty for many beneficiaries. That complexity appears to result from a number of separate factors, including

- the inherently complicated nature of the Medicare program design;
- the differences in coverage from area to area for some new medical tests;
- the enormous number of rules and the exceptions to those rules;
- the limited response to complaints about errors;
- the difficulties in communication between Medicare and Medicare beneficiaries.

Organizations such as the Medicare Rights Center and the United Seniors Health Cooperative, and state-sponsored counseling programs, can offer advice, information, and help to consumers in dealing with specific Medicare problems.

10

Medigap and Secondary Health Insurance Policies

Medigap policies help Medicare beneficiaries pay for the Medicare deductible and co-insurance amounts and for certain other medical costs that are not covered by the traditional Medicare program. Given the limits of that traditional program, many people consider a Medigap policy to be essential.

Years ago, there was an enormous variety of Medicare-supplementary policies available, and confusion and possible duplication of coverage represented serious problems. Although some older Medicare-supplementary policies may still exist, federal regulations now provide for only ten standardized Medigap plans to be offered to Medicare beneficiaries. Each plan is labeled by a letter, A through J.

The process of standardizing Medigap plans has had a number of positive results. First, each type of Medigap plan is now identical, regardless of the company through which it is offered. Thus, although Plan A may be offered by four or five different insurers in a particular area, the plan provides the same benefits in each case. That makes it easier for Medicare beneficiaries to focus on such issues as coverage, premiums, and service when deciding which Medigap plan to purchase. Second, standardization makes it easier to avoid duplicate coverage, since the benefits offered by each Medigap plan are clearly outlined.

Each of the ten standardized plans has significant differences, and each plan offers a different level of coverage. Medigap plans may not necessarily cover pre-existing conditions for the first six months. Aside from that, however, all of the plans (A through J) provide at least some coverage for co-insurance in terms of hospital stays and doctor's bills that are covered by Medicare.

Medigap Plans A and B are considered basic plans and offer very limited coverage. Plans H, I, and J provide the widest degree of coverage. Plan A primarily provides coverage for the co-insurance amount for hospitalization and the co-insurance amount for outpatient treatment under Medicare: Part B, amounts that are not generally covered by the traditional Medicare program. Plan B also provides some coverage for the hospital deductible amount.

Plan C includes coverage for the co-insurance amount for treatment in a skilled nursing facility, for the Medicare: Part B deductible, and for some emergency care outside of the United States, once a special deductible has been met. Plans D and G provide some coverage for home health care under certain conditions following an illness, accident, or surgery. That may include coverage for a brief period of time for home-based health care related to such activities of daily living as getting dressed and bathing.

Plans F, G, I, and J also offer coverage for Medicare excess charges, the additional 15% above the Medicare allowable amount that a provider who does not accept assignment may charge. Plans E and J offer limited coverage for certain types of preventive medical care. Plans H, I, and J provide coverage for a percentage of the cost of prescription medications. Plans H and I cover up to $1,250 per year in prescription costs; Plan J covers up to $3,000 per year (See Table 15).

There are other important differences between these Medigap plans, as well. A number of organizations offer booklets that explain those differences in detail (See Appendix B). The Department of Insurance or the Division on Aging in your state may also offer advice and information on Medigap plans.

It's important to be aware that not all Medigap plans are available in all states. However, Plan A is generally available throughout the United States, and most states allow a number of different Medigap policies to be offered by insurers in addition to Plan A. All ten plans are available to Medicare beneficiaries in some states.

In addition, you may be able to purchase a type of policy called **Medicare Select.** While Medicare Select is not one of the ten standardized Medigap policies discussed above, it fulfills some of the same functions. However, unlike the ten standardized Medigap policies, Medicare Select is based on a managed care approach.

Medigap plans sold in three states—Minnesota, Wisconsin, and Massachusetts—may not adhere specifically to any of the ten standardized plans. The Medigap program in those states pre-dates the federal standardization of Medigap insurance, and was thus allowed to continue in force after the federal program was put into effect. Check with your state Department of Insurance or Division on Aging to determine which Medigap policies are available in your state.

If you are about to enroll in Part B of the traditional Medicare plan and you are unable to afford a Medigap policy, the federal government may be able to provide some help. For example, the **Qualified Medicare Beneficiary** program (**QMB**) and the **Selected Low-Income Medicare Beneficiary** program (**SLMB**) may pay for specific Medicare costs under certain conditions.

For eligible individuals, the Qualified Medicare Beneficiary program may provide payment for Medicare deductibles, co-insurance amounts, and premiums. The Selected Low-Income Medicare Beneficiary program may pay Medicare: Part B premiums. Eligibility depends on income and assets. The basic difference between the two programs in terms of eligibility is that the Qualified Medicare Beneficiary program is available to individuals whose income is below the poverty level and whose assets are limited, while the Selected Low-Income Medicare Beneficiary program is available to individuals whose income is slightly above the poverty level. (See Appendix B for a list of booklets that describe these programs in detail.)

Table 15
Standardized Medigap Plans

Type of Plan	Coverage
Medigap Plan A	Coverage for co-insurance for hospitalization and doctors' bills
Medigap Plan B	Also provides coverage for hospital deductible
Medigap Plan C	Coverage for the co-insurance amount for treatment in a skilled nursing facility, for the Medicare: Part B deductible, and for some emergency care outside of the United States
Medigap Plan D	Coverage for some home health care
Medigap Plan E	Coverage for some preventive care
Medigap Plan F	Coverage for excess Medicare charges
Medigap Plan G	Coverage for excess Medicare charges and for some home health care
Medigap Plan H	Coverage for a percentage of prescription medications, up to $1,250 a year
Medigap Plan I	Coverage for a percentage of prescription medications, up to $1,250 a year

Table 15 (Continued)

Type of Plan	Coverage
Medigap Plan J	Coverage for a percentage of prescription medications, up to $3,000 a year
Medicare Select	While not technically one of the ten standardized Medigap policies, Medicare Select provides coverage by means of a managed care approach
Qualified Medicare Beneficiary (QMB) program	While not technically a standardized Medigap policy, the QMB program provides coverage for Medicare deductibles, co-insurance amounts, and premiums for eligible individuals whose income is below the poverty line and whose assets are limited
Selected Low-Income Medicare Beneficiary (SLMB) program	While not technically a standardized Medigap policy, the SLMB program provides coverage for Part B premiums for eligible individuals whose income is just above the poverty line

Note: All Medigap plans provide some coverage for the co-insurance amount for hospitalization and doctors' bills under Medicare: Part A and Part B.

It's important to research the various Medigap plans carefully before making a decision. Current regulations guarantee a choice of plans to senior citizens only during the first six months after enrolling in Medicare: Part B. Although the rules differ from state to state, that guarantee generally refers only to senior citizens, not to individuals who are under the age of 65 and who are covered by Medicare as a result of a disability.

If you choose a Medigap policy and then decide that you've made an error, you generally have the right to cancel the policy within the first thirty days. In that case, you may receive a refund of premiums. If you continue the policy beyond that thirty day period, you can still cancel the policy at any point. However, if you cancel your Medigap policy after the first six months, there is no guarantee that you will be able to purchase the policy of your choice in the future.

Under current rules, if you purchase a Medigap policy and decide to continue it on a permanent basis, the insurer cannot generally cancel it as long as you continue to pay the premiums on time. However, that rule applies only to the new standardized Medigap policies, not necessarily to policies issued prior to 1992. If you have an older policy, you are not required to switch to a standardized policy.

Although Medigap policies are clearly important for individuals who are covered by the traditional Medicare plan, Medigap policies do have one serious limitation: They may not provide reimbursement for a service or for medical equipment that Medicare does not consider to be a covered expense. However, some secondary insurance plans—employer-sponsored group health insurance plans that continue in place after retirement and that act as Medicare supplements—may provide benefits in such situations. In some cases, secondary insurance plans may provide reimbursement of up to 80% of the cost of such services or medical equipment. They may also pay for a percentage of the cost of prescription medications and of other items that are not generally covered under the traditional Medicare program.

For example, let's say that a Medicare beneficiary has developed severe arthritis, is unable to walk more than a block or so because of pain and joint inflammation, and needs a wheelchair for longer distances. Since the arthritis has also affected her arms and shoulders, making it impossible for her to handle a manual wheelchair, a power chair or an electric scooter is necessary. In order to qualify for reimbursement under Medicare, her doctor would generally have to be able to certify that her condition made the use of a wheelchair medically necessary, and that it would not be medically possible for her to make use of a manual wheelchair.

In addition, the doctor would also need to be able to certify that she required the wheelchair for use in the house. Since the individual in this case is able to walk a block, she would probably not meet Medicare's definition of medical necessity. Thus, she would not qualify for reimbursement for the purchase of a power wheelchair or an electric scooter. If the qualifications for reimbursement for a power wheelchair or electric scooter are not met according to Medicare standards, a Medigap policy would probably not provide reimbursement either.

However, a secondary health insurance policy might include a much wider definition of medical necessity. In some cases, a secondary health insurance policy might provide for reimbursement of up to 80% of the cost of the power wheelchair or electric scooter—assuming it provides for coordination-of-benefits with Medicare on an 80/20 basis—even though Medicare did not consider the wheelchair to be a covered expense. Since a power wheelchair may cost as much as $20,000—depending on the particular wheelchair and on the accessories—the difference in reimbursement between a Medigap policy and a secondary insurance policy would be highly significant in a situation such as this.

SUMMARY

Many people consider a Medigap policy to be essential for Medicare benefiaries who are covered by the traditional Medicare program. There are now ten standardized Medigap policies available, labeled A through J. Plan A offers the least coverage; plans H, I, and J offer the most coverage. Individuals in some states may also be eligible for Medicare Select, a Medicare-supplementary policy based on a managed care approach.

Individuals who are unable to afford a Medigap policy may be able to qualify for benefits under either the Qualified Medicare Beneficiary program or the Selected Low-Income Medicare Beneficiary program. Those programs may pay for specific Medicare costs under certain conditions. Although they are not technically considered standardized Medigap policies, these programs provide important economic benefits for eligible individuals.

Medigap policies are of enormous importance in many cases. However, secondary insurance policies that act as supplements to Medicare can offer significant advantages. Since such policies may include a different definition of medical necessity, secondary health insurance policies may provide coverage for treatments, services, or medical equipment in situations where such coverage might not be available under a Medigap policy.

11

Medicare HMOs

As part of the movement toward managed care, the federal government recently began to allow Medicare beneficiaries to obtain benefits through **Medicare HMOs** instead of through the traditional Medicare plan. These HMOs are designed specifically for Medicare beneficiaries who are enrolled in both Medicare: Part A and Medicare: Part B.

Medicare HMOs are paid by the government on the basis of either a **cost-based contract** or a **risk-based contract.** Under a cost-based contract, the federal government's payments to the HMO are based on the actual costs. Under a risk-based contract, the federal government pays a flat fee for each Medicare beneficiary enrolled in the HMO. That fee is determined statistically on the basis of an analysis of the average expenses of Medicare beneficiaries in the area in which the HMO operates, and may thus differ from area to area. At this point, the overwhelming majority of Medicare HMOs operate under risk-based contracts.

Medicare HMOs may offer important benefits to Medicare beneficiaries. While the traditional Medicare plan allows beneficiaries to choose their own doctors, hospitals, and testing centers, there are significant limitations in terms of coverage and deductibles. In contrast, in addition to providing coverage for the standard types of Medicare benefits, Medicare HMOs may also provide some benefits for services that are not covered under the traditional Medicare plan. Those additional benefits may include coverage for prescription medications, hearing aids, eyeglasses, and such preventive services as vaccinations and annual physical exams. The specific benefits differ from one Medicare HMO to another.

However, Medicare HMOs generally have a series of specialized rules that participants must follow in order to obtain maximum benefits. First, some Medicare HMOs may provide full coverage only if the participant makes use of medical providers who are part of the plan network. Second, access to medical specialists or to expensive medical tests may be determined by the gatekeeper, the participant's primary care physician. That includes access to specialists such as neurologists, rheumotologists, and psychiatrists, as well as access to tests such as CAT scans and MRIs. Finally, some Medicare HMO's may provide coverage outside of the HMO's geographic area only for emergency treatment. (See Table 16 for a comparison of the traditional Medicare plan and Medicare HMOs.)

Although all Medicare HMOs have certain features in common, there may also be important differences between them. For example, some Medicare HMOs may provide reimbursement for both emergency care and urgent care outside the HMO's geographic area. In addition, some Medicare HMOs now offer a special option—at additional cost—that allows participants to occasionally see medical providers outside of the provider network and still qualify for some reimbursement. That option is generally referred to as a **Point-of-Service** or **POS** Option.

In some cases, a Medigap policy may not be necessary when a Medicare beneficiary joins a Medicare HMO, since the coverage provided by the Medigap policy may simply duplicate coverage offered by the HMO. Canceling a Medigap policy may save a good deal of money. However, if you join a Medicare HMO and then cancel your Medigap policy, it's important to be aware that there is no guarantee that you will be able to enroll in a new Medigap policy of your choice if you decide to return to the traditional Medicare plan.

Table 16
Comparison of the Traditional Medicare Plan and Medicare HMOs

Issue	Traditional Medicare Plan	Medicare HMOs
Coverage for standard types of care such as doctors' visits and tests	Yes	Yes
Need for Medigap plan	Yes	May not be necessary
Need to obtain approval for expensive tests or consultations with a specialist	No	Yes
Coverage for prescription medications	No	Yes, in many cases
Coverage for eyeglasses, hearing aids	No	Yes, in many cases
Coverage for preventive care	No (except for situations such as coverage for certain vaccines)	Yes

Note: Coverage for some of these services may also be available through a Medigap plan.

The rules that deal with the right of a Medicare beneficiary to choose a specific Medigap policy differ from state to state. Given that situation, it may be a good idea for Medicare beneficiaries who have a Medigap policy when they join a Medicare HMO to maintain that policy temporarily until they are certain that the Medicare HMO will fully meet their needs and that they want to remain in the HMO on a permanent basis. During that period of time, the Medicare beneficiary will have an opportunity to evaluate the coverage offered by both the HMO and the Medigap policy, and can make a logical determination in terms of whether the coverage offered by the Medigap policy is likely to be beneficial in the long run.

Many members of Medicare HMOs report a high level of satisfaction with the program in which they're enrolled. However, there have also been reports of problems. The government is currently in the process of reviewing the possibility of developing a system for evaluating Medicare HMOs. If that system is established, it should make it much easier to decide whether a Medicare HMO is appropriate for you. Since it's likely to be several years before the system is in place, you'll need to rely on your own research in the meantime. Before making any decision, it's essential to compare several Medicare HMOs, to discuss the rules with program representatives, and to talk with HMO members about their experiences.

SUMMARY

The decision of whether to stay with the traditional Medicare plan or to join a Medicare HMO is an important one. The question of which HMO to join is equally important. Before making any decision, it's essential for Medicare beneficiaries to research a variety of Medicare HMOs and to compare those choices with the advantages and disadvantages of staying with the traditional Medicare plan.

Part IV
SPECIALIZED SITUATIONS

12

Extending Coverage through COBRA, the Portability Act, and Conversion Options

There are a number of circumstances—including job changes, divorce, and retirement—in which an individual might wish to continue an existing health insurance policy after coverage under that policy would normally end. At present, there are three mechanisms through which that goal can be achieved: **COBRA,** the **Portability and Accountability Act**, and **conversion options.**

COBRA

COBRA is an acronym. The letters stand for **Consolidated Omnibus Budget Reconciliation Act,** a law that deals with a number of different issues, including the continuation of health insurance. Under certain conditions, COBRA regulations allow for the continuation of health insurance benefits for up to 18 months for eligible employees and for up to 36 months for their eligible dependents.

COBRA regulations that relate to private health insurance plans are administered on a national level by the Pension and Welfare Benefits Administration of the United States Department of Labor. COBRA regulations that relate to health insurance plans sponsored by state or municipal government agencies are administered by the United States Public Health Service (See Appendix B). While these national offices set basic rules and deal with specific complaints, they do not provide health insurance. Instead, COBRA allows for an extension of existing health insurance policies.

Once a health insurance policy has been extended under COBRA, claims may still be processed by the previous insurer, and claim rules will remain the same. However, the premium will be based on the cost of the existing health insurance policy plus a 2% fee. That rate is generally stated as "102% of the premium." The premium, of course, varies from policy to policy. You can obtain the exact premium for continuing your health insurance policy under COBRA from your employer's benefits office.

The extension of health insurance benefits under COBRA may be particularly useful in situations in which

- an individual has retired and is no longer covered by an employer-sponsored group health insurance plan, but still has a few months to wait until eligibility for Medicare occurs;
- an individual is between jobs and wants to continue health insurance coverage temporarily;
- a child is no longer covered under a family's health insurance plan because of age, but is not yet eligible for health insurance through his own employment;
- a spouse is no longer eligible for health insurance coverage due to divorce or to the death of the employee.

The length of time for which a COBRA extension is available depends on the **qualifying event,** the reason for which the COBRA extension is required. If the qualifying event is the loss of health insurance coverage due to termination of employment or a reduction in hours, an eligible employee may be entitled to a continuation of health insurance benefits for up to 18 months.

If the employee has a disability, it may be possible to increase that extension by an additional 11 months, for a total of 29 months. However, the individual's disability must generally meet the definition set by the Social Security Act in order to qualify for the additional extension. In addition, the premium may increase significantly during the extension period, up to a maximum of 150% of the cost of the health insurance itself. In some cases, the 11 month extension may end immediately if the person becomes eligible for Medicare.

If the qualifying event is a divorce or the death of the employee, eligible dependents may be entitled to a continuation of health insurance benefits under COBRA for up to 36 months. If the qualifying event is the loss of health insurance for a child because the child has reached the age at which he is no longer eligible for such insurance as a dependent under his parents' policy, he may also be entitled to a continuation of health insurance benefits under COBRA for up to 36 months.

The procedure for continuing health insurance benefits under COBRA is fairly simple. A form that allows for a continuation of health insurance should be sent out automatically by the insurer or the employer when a qualifying event occurs. Generally, all the consumer needs to do at that point is to fill out the form, write out a check, and send it to the address printed on the form.

If you wish to continue health insurance benefits under COBRA, and you have not received a form, you can obtain one from your employer's benefits office. Canceling a COBRA extension is just as simple: Whenever a check is not submitted, coverage automatically ends.

However, there are some circumstances in which COBRA regulations may not apply, or may not be helpful. For example, if you work for a company that has fewer than 20 employees, you and/or your dependents may not be eligible to continue your health insurance benefits under COBRA, even if you might otherwise have qualified for a continuation of such benefits.

In addition, specialized rules apply in situations in which health insurance is provided through an HMO. HMOs are generally centered in a particular geographic area, and coverage may be provided only for emergency services outside of that area. Thus, if you lose your job and move to another area of the country, you may not be eligible to continue your HMO coverage under COBRA.

However, if your employer offers a traditional health insurance plan, you may be able to switch to that plan during an open enrollment period before you leave your job. Once you've made that switch, you may be able to apply for an extension of the traditional plan under COBRA when you move. If it's not possible to switch to a traditional policy, COBRA rules may not be helpful. COBRA regulations do not require a company to create a new insurance plan in order to meet the needs of an employee who is moving to a new area.

There are a number of other technical rules and exceptions that exist in relation to COBRA. You can obtain additional information by talking with a representative at the benefits office of your current or former employer, or by calling or writing to a benefits advisor at the Pension and Welfare Benefits Administration of the United States Department of Labor. If your health insurance is provided by a state or municipal government agency, you can write instead to the United States Public Health Service, which has jurisdiction over the implementation of COBRA regulations in such situations (See Appendix B).

One common problem of which you should be aware is that some insurance companies may issue a new identification number when an individual continues health insurance under COBRA. However, that identification number may not be cross-referenced to the individual's previous identification number. Thus, if you continue your health insurance under COBRA, you may find that claims filed under your previous identification number will be rejected on the grounds that your insurance coverage has been terminated. If that occurs, the solution is generally to call your insurer, find out your new identification number, and re-file the claims under that number.

THE PORTABILITY AND ACCOUNTABILITY ACT

Although continuing a health insurance policy through COBRA can be very helpful in many situations, it may not always be the best approach. In some cases, it may be more appropriate to continue health insurance through the Portability and Accountability Act, particularly when changing jobs. The Portability and Accountability Act states that under certain conditions, an eligible individual who has been covered by health insurance can switch jobs and join a new health insurance plan without any limitations in terms of coverage for pre-existing conditions. In many cases, that may make it possible for an individual to consider changing jobs without worrying about health insurance issues.

In order to qualify for the benefits offered under the act, an individual who is in the process of changing jobs must have been enrolled in a previous employer-sponsored group health insurance plan for at least 12 months. In addition, the switch from the previous employer-sponsored group health insurance plan to the new employer-sponsored group health insurance plan must occur within 63 days. However, if the switch is from an employer-sponsored group health insurance plan to an individual policy, the individual must have been previously covered by a health insurance plan for at least 18 months. In addition, the individual must first exhaust benefits available under COBRA, Medicare, Medicaid, or other health insurance plans, before applying for an individual policy.

According to the act, if an individual continues health insurance under a previous group health insurance plan through COBRA and then transfers to an individual health insurance policy, the transfer from COBRA to the new individual policy must occur within 63 days, as well. These provisions of the Portability and Accountability Act took effect on July 1, 1997. Credit for the 12 or 18 months of prior enrollment in a health insurance plan began as of July of 1996. However, in some cases, these rules may be superseded by state laws.

CONVERSION OPTIONS

Neither COBRA nor the Portability and Accountability Act is likely to be of much value in cases in which an individual has reached the lifetime benefit maximum provided for in a health insurance policy. However, exercising a **conversion option**—an option included in some group health insurance plans—may be of enormous value in such situations. Exercising a conversion option allows an individual to convert from a group plan to an individual policy, thus providing for the possibility of a series of additional benefits.

For example, let's assume that an individual has a serious disease or condition—cancer, AIDS (acquired immune deficiency syndrome), MS (multiple sclerosis), a serious heart problem—that has resulted in extremely high medical bills over a period of years, and that the individual's group health insurance plan has a lifetime benefit maximum of $250,000. If the individual's total medical expenses are approaching that lifetime benefit maximum—for example, if they have reached $225,000—the individual may soon reach a point where he will officially continue to be covered by the health insurance plan, but no additional benefits will be available. However, if the group plan allows for conversion to an individual policy, acting on that option may allow for significant additional benefits.

Although the exercise of a conversion option may not represent a policy extension from a technical point of view, since the original policy is still officially available, on a practical basis it may serve the same purpose. The amount of reimbursement available after the conversion to an individual policy takes place depends on the particular policy. In some cases, conversion to an individual policy may provide a wide range of additional benefits. In other cases, both the benefits and the lifetime benefit maximum may be quite limited.

If you have a serious disease or condition and your medical bills are approaching the lifetime benefit maximum under your health insurance plan, check with your insurer or with your employer's benefits representative to determine if a conversion option is available. If such an option is available under the rules of your health insurance plan, check to determine what specific benefits will be available once the conversion from the group plan to an individual policy occurs.

SUMMARY

In some cases, a health insurance policy can be extended through COBRA, the Portability and Accountability Act, and the exercise of the conversion option offered by some group health insurance plans.

Using these mechanisms can make it possible for an individual to continue a health insurance policy for an extended period in situations in which the policy would normally end, without worrying about exclusions for pre-existing conditions or an immediate loss of benefits. Those situations may include divorce, changing jobs, or reaching the lifetime benefit maximum provided for in a health insurance policy.

13

Programs for Children and Adults with Disabilities and Special Health Care Needs

Children and adults with disabilities or special health care needs may sometimes find that they have difficulty in obtaining health insurance, or that their medical needs are not fully met by their existing individual or group health insurance policies. In such cases, coverage for medical treatment or durable medical equipment may be available through Medicaid, through other programs sponsored by state and federal agencies, or through alternate sources of funding.

MEDICAID

Some children with disabilities and special health care needs may be eligible for health insurance coverage through **Medicaid.** Medicaid is a government-sponsored program designed to provide health insurance for eligible children with disabilities and for eligible individuals whose incomes fall below the poverty line. In the case of children with disabilities, eligibility is determined partly on the basis of family income.

Currently, Medicaid serves as an essential part of the American system of health insurance. However, it unfortunately appears to suffer from the same complex, fragmented, approach that seems to serve as the basis for the overall health insurance system in America. For example, Medicaid originated as a federal program and continues to be partially funded by the federal government. However, each state is given the authority to develop many of the rules under which the particular program will operate within that state. Thus, while federal regulations provide for a core of basic services in all states, including doctors' visits and hospital care, individual states can determine whether or not to offer certain optional aspects of the program. As a result, the Medicaid program may differ significantly from state to state.

MEDICAID WAIVERS

The Medicaid program may also differ from state to state as a result of the Medicaid waiver system. Federal law currently allows individual states to request specific **Medicaid waivers.** Each waiver exempts the particular state from a set of federal Medicaid regulations and/or specific restrictions. Some waivers relate to the way in which services are delivered and deal with issues such as coverage through Medicaid HMOs and other types of managed care programs. Other Medicaid waivers are part of the home and community-based waiver system, and relate to eligibility for particular services.

A number of waivers have already been established and may be applied for by any state Medicaid office. Proposals for new waivers can be developed by an individual state at any time. Two established Medicaid waivers—the **Katie Beckett** waiver and the **Traumatic Brain Injury** waiver—serve as illustrations of waivers that relate to eligibility for services.

The Katie Beckett waiver was developed in the early 1980s. The rule at that time was that Medicaid generally included the parents' income in determining a disabled child's eligibility for benefits if the child lived at home. However, Medicaid did not include the parents' income if the child was hospitalized or institutionalized for an extended period.

As a result, children like Katie Beckett—who was on a ventilator in a hospital—were sometimes eligible for continued Medicaid coverage only if they remained in the hospital, even though home care would have been more appropriate and far less expensive. In many cases, the lack of Medicaid coverage for home-based care in such situations made it economically impossible for families to provide the medical equipment and the medical services necessary to care for a child at home.

The problem was eventually solved through the creation of a special Medicaid waiver. Under the terms of the waiver, Medicaid can provide for home-based care in situations in which a child is covered by Medicaid while in a hospital or an institution, is medically able to return home, but can do so only if the family has the economic help and support it needs to purchase the necessary medical equipment and to provide care.

Since that time, the Katie Beckett waiver has helped a number of children in such situations, children who would otherwise have been forced to stay in hospitals or institutions on a permanent basis. Katie Beckett waivers have now been developed in most states, although the particular regulations and the populations they serve may differ significantly from state to state.

The traumatic brain injury waiver permits a state to spend Medicaid funds for community-based transition programs—including rehabilitation programs and case management—for individuals who have experienced severe brain injuries. Community-based transition programs for people with brain injuries may be far less expensive than inpatient care, and may allow individuals to benefit from the help and support of friends and family members. At this point, services under traumatic brain injury waivers are available in a number of states. However, the programs may differ significantly from state to state. Since the traumatic brain injury waiver has already been established, any state can apply for a similar waiver whenever it wishes.

One of the newest Medicaid waivers involves programs that provide coverage for specific types of long-term care for senior citizens with disabilities or illnesses. Such waivers may eventually allow some senior citizens in those states that have been granted the waiver the opportunity to reside in assisted living facilities rather than in nursing homes. (See Chapter 14 for a further discussion of Medicaid waivers that relate to assisted living for senior citizens.)

Each of these waivers is important. However, the specific services provided by each waiver are available only to Medicaid recipients in those states in which the particular waiver has been adopted. If you or a family member are unable to obtain needed care because your state Medicaid program does not provide coverage for the necessary services—unlike programs in other states—it may be possible to work with the state Medicaid office to develop an appropriate waiver. The key to ensuring the development of a Medicaid waiver or trying to obtain changes in state Medicaid rules is generally to seek the help of local or national advocacy or support groups, disability rights organizations, and legislative representatives. Advocacy groups, support groups, and disability rights organizations often have the knowledge and the skills needed to work with the state and federal Medicaid program to develop an application for a new waiver. Legislative representatives have the authority to hold hearings to discuss proposed changes in state Medicaid regulations.

MEDICAID APPEALS AND ELIGIBILITY RULES

If you or a family member are unable to obtain needed care because your application for Medicaid has been rejected, and you think the application should have been approved under the existing rules of your state, it's important to make use of the Medicaid appeals process as soon as possible. Although the appeals system differs from state to state, the process generally includes an opportunity to appeal to a **neutral hearing officer.** While an appeal may result in a decision to grant Medicaid benefits, there is no guarantee of success.

There are a number of helpful booklets available on the issue of Medicaid appeals (See Appendix B). If you need more specific advice about a Medicaid appeal, the local Legal Services Office may also be able to help. You can locate the nearest office by calling the National Legal Aid and Defender Association (See Appendix B).

The local Bar Association may be able to provide information on the nearest Legal Services Office, as well. The Bar Association may also be able to refer you to the local office of the Protection and Advocacy Service, which may be particularly helpful on Medicaid eligibility issues or claim denials if the situation involves a child with a disability. There are also private organizations, including a number of disability law centers, that can provide help and advice with Medicaid-related issues (See Appendix B).

If you are considering applying for Medicaid for yourself or a family member, and there are assets that may affect eligibility, you should be aware that there are a number of laws that may relate to such assets. Thus, it's important to review your situation carefully with an attorney or with an agency such as the Protection and Advocacy Service or Legal Services before making any decisions about assets.

RECENT CHANGES IN MEDICAID RULES

Once the issue of eligibility has been resolved, and an individual is covered by Medicaid, it's important to understand the program rules in order to obtain appropriate benefits. Unfortunately, those rules are complex and are often difficult to comprehend. In addition, the rules under which the Medicaid program operates have changed significantly over the years.

One change that directly affects children with disabilities involves the establishment of the **Early Periodic Screening, Diagnosis, and Treatment** (**EPSDT**) program. EPSDT provides for a periodic medical screening for children with disabilities. In many cases, a medical need identified as a result of that screening may be eligible for Medicaid coverage as long as it is covered under federal rules, even if that need would not ordinarily be covered under the rules of the particular state's Medicaid program. The *EPSDT Reference Law Manual* describes current EPSDT regulations. That manual is available through the National Health Law Program (See Appendix B). Although the manual is technical in nature, it may be helpful to parents of children with disabilities, since it is highly specific regarding childrens' rights to medical services.

Another more recent change involves the shift to managed care. **Medicaid HMOs** (Health Maintenance Organizations) are rapidly becoming an important part of the Medicaid system in many states. In some ways, the development of Medicaid HMOs may make it easier for Medicaid recipients to obtain medical care, since there is a specific network of providers available to meet their needs. Thus, patients may avoid unnecessary trips to the hospital emergency room.

Medicaid HMOs may also allow medical tests and services to be delivered in a more organized manner, since all medical care is generally coordinated by the individual's primary care physician. Medicaid HMOs may offer coverage for preventive services, as well. In addition, the establishment of Medicaid HMOs may provide significant cost savings for the government.

However, the transition to managed care may create a great deal of confusion for some Medicaid recipients. For example, it may take time for each Medicaid recipient to choose a primary care physician and to learn the somewhat complex rules of managed care.

Managed care programs generally require prior approval from the primary care physician before a participant visits a hospital emergency room—except perhaps for a serious emergency—consults a specialist, or schedules medical tests. Such programs may also require that participants use only network providers. It may take time for some Medicaid recipients to adjust to the new rules.

MEDICARE

Although people generally think of Medicare as a health insurance program for senior citizens, in some cases Medicare is also available to help meet the needs of people with disabilities.

For example, under certain conditions Medicare coverage may be available to individuals under age 65 who become disabled and are no longer able to work. Coverage may also be available to both children and adults who have End-Stage Renal Disease (ESRD) and require kidney dialysis treatments. In such cases, Medicare can be of enormous importance in providing coverage for the cost of medical care.

OTHER LAWS AND PROGRAMS

Although Medicaid and Medicare serve as essential sources of health insurance coverage for many people with disabilities, there are other laws that may offer help, as well. For example, some children and adults with spina bifida may qualify for benefits under the federal **Spina Bifida-Agent Orange Benefits Act,** passed in September of 1996. The act covers children and adults with certain types of spina bifida whose biological parents were exposed to Agent Orange during the Vietnam conflict. The Spina Bifida-Agent Orange Benefits Act may provide for health care and rehabilitation for eligible individuals. The law is scheduled to become effective during the fall of 1997.

In addition, the federal **Mental Health Parity Act,** passed in September of 1996, offers help for individuals with mental illnesses who are covered by group health insurance plans. (See Chapter 4 for further information on federal and state parity laws).

Many people with disabilities may be covered by private health insurance policies, as well. In some cases, a private health insurance policy may serve as the primary insurer, with Medicaid as the secondary insurer.

However, it's sometimes difficult for people with disabilities to obtain health insurance. There are private organizations that offer health insurance programs that are designed specifically for people with disabilities. For example, The Arc—a national organization on mental retardation—offers a group health insurance plan designed to meet the needs of individuals with disabilities who are between the ages of 10 and 65 (See Appendix B for further information). However, there is no guarantee of acceptance in The Arc plan. Rather, the medical history and insurability of each applicant is individually evaluated. The Arc plan is offered on a national basis, and is available to residents of most states.

If your family is covered by a private health insurance policy, it's important to be aware that some private health insurance policies may allow for a permanent extension of health insurance for a child with a disability in certain cases, even after the point at which the child would usually be excluded from continued coverage on the basis of age. Check with your insurance company to determine the rules of your policy in regard to the continuation of health insurance coverage for a child with a disability.

While private health insurance policies may offer important benefits for people with disabilities, there may also be a number of limitations in terms of coverage. For example, while power wheelchairs are generally covered by health insurance policies, wheelchair lifts, ramps, and other wheelchair-related equipment may not be covered.

Although some states have passed laws dealing with health insurance coverage for specific items—for example, for infant formula for children with specific types of disabilities who are unable to digest standard foods—those laws apply only in certain situations and only in the states that have enacted such legislation. Private health insurance policies in states that have not enacted such legislation might not provide any coverage for items such as infant formula. If your child is affected by that limitation or by other rules or limitations, the solution may be to work with an advocacy or support group, a disability rights organization, or with legislative representatives to try to change the laws in your state.

ALTERNATE SOURCES OF FUNDING

There are a variety of situations in which neither Medicaid, Medicare, or private health insurance policies are likely to offer coverage for important services or equipment. Fortunately, there are public and private programs and agencies that may be able to provide help in such cases, particularly in terms of meeting the needs of a child with a disability.

For example, certain services for a child with a disability who is attending school may be available through the local public school district. In some cases, a local public school district may consider providing such services as speech therapy and physical therapy for a child with a disability, and may also consider providing help with the purchase of an augmentative communications device, a hearing aid, or other types of medical equipment. To qualify for help through a local school district, you need to be able to demonstrate that the particular equipment is directly related to the child's education. In addition, the need for the equipment must generally be listed in the child's **IEP (Individualized Education Program).**

The state **Division of Vocational Rehabilitation Services (DVRS)** may be able to provide help for an older child with a disability who is beginning to prepare for employment. There are DVRS offices in each state. The Division of Vocational Rehabilitation Services may be able to provide vocational testing, counseling, and education related to employment. DVRS may also be able to make referrals to agencies that provide services related to supported employment programs and job placement. In addition, DVRS may be able to help purchase equipment or make modifications that are directly related to employment. For further information, contact your local state Division of Vocational Rehabilitation Services office.

There are also programs designed to help families purchase used, inexpensive, medical equipment that may not be covered by Medicaid or by private health insurance policies. For example, many of the **Tech Act** programs established under the 1988 federal **Technology-Related Assistance for Individuals with Disabilities Act** offer used durable medical equipment. Such equipment may incude wheelchairs, specially equipped vans, lifts, ramps, computers with specialized equipment, TTYs (teletype writers), augmentative communications devices, walkers, crutches, and speech synthesizers.

There are Tech Act programs in each state, although they may operate under different names. In New Jersey, the Tech Act program is known as TARP (Technology Assistive Resource Program). In Indiana, the program is called ATTAIN (Accessing Technology Through Awareness In Indiana), while in Oregon, the program is referred to as TALN (Technology Access For Life Needs).

RESNA (Rehabilitation Engineering and Assistive Technology Society of North America) serves as the technical consultant for Tech Act programs throughout the country. RESNA can provide a list of telephone numbers for the various state programs, and may also be able to offer information on the services available through each program (See Appendix B).

At present, there are two different types of used equipment programs available through Tech Act agencies: equipment exchange and equipment recycling. Equipment exchange programs match people who have agreed to sell or donate durable medical equipment with people who need such equipment. The equipment is usually owned by individuals and generally remains in the individual's home until it is purchased.

The following states currently have equipment exchange programs: Alaska, Arkansas, Delaware, Georgia, Illinois, Indiana, Iowa, Kentucky, Minnesota, Mississippi, Montana, Nebraska, Nevada, New Hampshire, New Jersey, New York, North Carolina, Oregon, Pennsylvania, South Carolina, Utah, Vermont, Virginia, and West Virginia.

Equipment recycling programs involve equipment that is usually held in a storage area operated by the Tech Act program or by other organizations. Much of the equipment may have been donated by corporations, and it often includes computers and computer-related products.

The following states currently operate equipment recycling programs: Georgia, Illinois, Kentucky, Mississippi, Nevada, New Hampshire, New York, and Oklahoma. Some of those state programs focus only on computers and computer-related equipment. New programs are in the process of being developed in other states.

In some areas, the Tech Act agency may operate the equipment exchange or recycling programs directly. In other areas, the programs may be operated with other organizations.

It's important to be aware that although many of the items available through the Tech Act programs may be relatively inexpensive, there are generally no guarantees in terms of the equipment. That can be particularly important if you're considering purchasing an expensive item such as a power wheelchair, a wheelchair lift, or a specially equipped computer, where it may not be possible to thoroughly examine or test all of the electronic or computer circuits.

Support for the purchase of medical equipment may also be available through a private grant. For example, the Disabled Children's Relief Fund offers grants that are designed to help families purchase wheelchairs, prosthetic devices, TTYs, or other kinds of medical equipment for children with disabilities (See Appendix B). Preference is generally given to individuals who need medical equipment that is not eligible for coverage through health insurance (See Table 17).

Local fraternal or service organizations may also help parents purchase medical equipment for children with disabilities. Organizations such as the **Telephone Pioneers**—a group made up of volunteers from various telephone companies—may provide help with disability-related architectural or engineering projects (See Appendix B).

The local Independent Living Center may have information about other volunteer groups or other local sources of funding to meet the needs of children with disabilities. In addition, state governments offer a variety of special programs for children and adults with disabilities. In some states, that may include programs designed to provide health insurance, medical equipment, or help with the cost of prescription medications.

Unfortunately, it's often difficult to find out about such state programs because they may be offered through different agencies in different states, and may be offered through a number of different agencies within a particular state.

Table 17
Alternate Sources of Funding for Equipment and Services for Children with Disabilities

Equipment or Service	Possible Source of Funds
Specially equipped computers, TTYs, augmentative communications devices	Tech Act programs (used medical equipment); state Division of Vocational Rehabilitation Services; various state agencies; Disabled Children's Relief Fund; local fraternal organizations; Independent Living Centers; local public school districts
Physical therapy, speech therapy	Local public school districts (for children of school age)
Wheelchairs (manual and power)	Tech Act programs (used durable medical equipment)
Ramps, modifications, or equipment related to wheelchair use	Tech Act programs (used durable medical equipment); Disabled Children's Relief Fund; local fraternal organizations; Independent Living Centers; Telephone Pioneers (construction; engineering)
Special equipment for wheelchair-users, including wheelchair lifts,and special seats	Local fraternal and service organizations; Tech Act programs (used durable medical equipment); Division of Vocational Rehabilitation Services

In some states, programs designed to help purchase medical equipment for children with disabilities may be available through the state Department of Health, the Division of Vocational Rehabilitation Services, the Division of Developmental Disabilities, or through another state agency. If you are unable to determine whether such funding programs are available in your state, or which state agency implements existing programs, the local office of the Protection and Advocacy Service or the local Independent Living Center may be able to help (See Appendix B).

Medications may be available through the "Prescription Drug Patient Assistance Program," sponsored by individual manufacturers of specific prescription medications. The program is intended to provide prescription medications for individuals who are unable to afford the cost of the medication.

Each manufacturer sets specific rules. Eligibility is usually determined on a case-by-case basis. The application must be made by the patient's physician (See Appendix B).

SUMMARY

Ideally, America will eventually devise an effective system through which children and adults with disabilities will have full access to the kinds of medical treatment, services, and equipment they need. In the meantime, it's essential to understand and make use of existing programs. At this point, programs that may provide health insurance coverage or funding for medical equipment and services for children with disabilities include Medicaid, Medicare, private health insurance policies, state programs, private organizations, and the public school system. Making use of the benefits offered through those programs will help ensure that children with disabilities have the opportunity to achieve their maximum potential.

14

Coverage for Long-term Care

Over the past century, the human life span has increased dramatically, offering an opportunity for people to live a rich, full life well into their seventies, eighties, and nineties. At the same time, that increased life-span may also mean that a large number of people are likely to require long-term care at some point in their lives, either at home, at an assisted living facility, in a skilled nursing facility, or in a nursing home.

Permanent care in a nursing home obviously needs to be seriously considered under certain circumstances, and may be essential in some situations. However, many senior citizens seem to feel that the ideal arrangement is to maintain maximum independence in their home community, whenever possible. Thus, when senior citizens become ill or disabled, their goal is often to make arrangements for long-term care to be provided at home.

In order to ensure that such an arrangement remains a possibility, long-term care needs to be available through an appropriate system of home health care services, local day care programs, and community-based support services. Unfortunately, our society has not yet made the adjustments that are necessary to ensure that coverage for such care is available for all senior citizens with disabilities or illnesses. At present, neither traditional health insurance policies, Medicare, or Medigap policies provide sufficient coverage in such situations.

HEALTH INSURANCE PLANS, MEDICARE, MEDIGAP

Traditional health insurance policies generally provide only limited coverage for home-based long-term care. Under certain conditions, Medicare may provide limited coverage for some types of home health care, including skilled nursing services, management of medications, physical therapy, and other related services. However, Medicare rules require that a doctor certify that there is a medical need for skilled home care. In addition, the care must generally be provided by a Medicare-certified agency, and the Medicare beneficiary must be considered home-bound.

Medicare may provide coverage for durable medical equipment, as well, and for treatment in a skilled nursing facility following a period of hospitalization. Medicare may also provide coverage for home-based hospice care for beneficiaries who are terminally ill. However, Medicare does not generally provide coverage for nursing home placements that primarily involve personal care.

Several of the standardized Medigap policies may also offer coverage for specific types of home health care for Medicare beneficiaries. (See Chapter 10 for additional information on Medigap policies.) Such coverage, though, is limited, and is generally available only if the individual has first met the Medicare requirements for home health care.

MEDICAID

For eligible individuals, Medicaid—a program sponsored by both the states and the federal government—may provide coverage for long-term care, including skilled nursing care. Medicaid may also provide coverage for many types of durable medical equipment related to home health care (e.g., wheelchairs, walkers, braces), and for care in a nursing home, even when the services offered primarily involve personal care.

In some states, Medicaid may also provide coverage for some aspects of specialized senior citizens' **day care pro-**

grams. Such coverage may be available to senior citizens with physical disabilities and cognitive impairments due to a stroke, Alzheimer's disease, or other conditions or illnesses. Day care programs may include a wide range of services, including meals, transportation, and recreational activities.

Some day care programs for senior citizens may also offer help in ensuring that medication is taken properly and may offer supportive services to care for diabetes, high blood pressure, and other chronic conditions. Some programs may also offer activities that are designed to maximize existing cognitive abilities. Day care programs for senior citizens may be of enormous importance to individuals who have chronic conditions or disabilities, and may make it possible for some senior citizens to continue to live active, satisfying lives while remaining in their homes and in the community.

However, many decisions regarding the types of services that are covered by Medicaid are made on the state level rather than on the federal level. Thus, the services that are available to Medicaid recipients differ significantly from state to state. For example, as we discussed earlier, the Medicaid programs in a number of states have received federal waivers that allow for coverage for some types of long-term care for eligible Medicaid recipients in an assisted living facility rather than in a nursing home.

Assisted living facilities may offer a wide range of services, depending on individual needs and on the particular program. Assisted living generally involves moving to a special apartment complex or residence. Depending on the situation, available services may include recreation programs, meals, housekeeping, medical and nursing services, and emergency services. Some individuals may need only minor supportive services, such as housekeeping and meals, while others may need the entire range of services, including medical and nursing care.

The availability of coverage for some types of care at an assisted living facility may offer an additional range of choices for senior citizens who require a more supportive program of long-term care than they can obtain at home, but who do not require nursing home care.

Those choices, though, are only available in states that have obtained the appropriate federal waivers. In addition, the programs may differ significantly in each state. Check with your state Medicaid office to determine whether your state has received a waiver related to coverage for assisted living facilities.

In all cases, Medicaid eligibility is dependent on meeting certain qualifications in regard to income and assets. Those eligibility requirements are set on the state level. Thus, the requirements may differ from state to state.

LONG-TERM CARE INSURANCE

The lack of universal health insurance coverage for long-term care, the Medicaid eligibility requirements, and the movement toward maximum independence for all people with illnesses or disabilities, makes careful planning for long-term care essential. That planning should begin as early as possible, long before a health emergency or crisis develops. In addition, since plans for long-term care may directly involve family members, and may affect taxes, wills, and a variety of other related issues, such planning should include discussions with family members, a financial advisor, and an attorney.

One aspect of that planning should be to consider the possibility of purchasing a long-term care insurance policy. Such policies are designed to provide coverage for long-term care—either in the home or in a specialized facility—under certain conditions.

The federal Portability and Accountability Act has triggered renewed interest in long-term care policies. The act includes a provision that may make it possible for premiums for such policies to be considered partly tax deductible in some cases. However, long-term care policies must meet certain federal standards in order to qualify under the provisions of the Portability and Accountability Act.

Choosing a long-term care policy can be complicated. One problem is that long-term care policies are not standardized. The advantages of standardization from the consumer's point of view can be seen by examining policies like Medigap that are already standardized, or by reviewing individual and small-employer health insurance plans in those states that now require standardization of such plans. One of the most important advantages is that standardized policies of a particular type are identical, regardless of which company issues them. In addition, each type of policy is usually labeled by letter for easy identification. That makes it easier for consumers to understand the policies, to compare coverage, premiums, and service, and to more easily avoid duplication of benefits.

The disadvantage of standardization is that it may not be possible to obtain coverage for a particular benefit or service that may be of concern to an individual, unless such coverage happens to be included in one of the standardized policies. If policies were not standardized, it might be possible to find a policy that does offer such coverage, or to find a company that would consider adding such coverage to the policy.

Given the current situation, long-term care policies should be carefully evaluated on an individual basis. That requires a great deal of time and research. One area that should be particularly researched relates to the costs involved. Although long-term care policies may provide important economic benefits, they may be expensive in some cases. Thus, it's essential to consider the question of how policy premiums will affect your economic situation, both now and in the future. In addition, you need to consider the costs as compared to the possible benefits.

Before making a decision, ask companies that issue long-term care insurance to send you copies of their policies. Review each of the policies carefully. It's important to determine exactly what types of care are covered or excluded, and the specific conditions under which coverage is available. In particular, make certain that the type of care with which you are most concerned is clearly covered. In addition to coverage designed to meet the needs of specific physical impairments or limitations, you may also want to make certain that the policy provides coverage for cognitive disorders due to a stroke or to conditions such as Alzheimer's Disease.

If your major concern is coverage for care in a nursing home—rather than coverage for home care, day care, or assisted living—it's important to consider policies that include provisions to cover possible increases in nursing home costs. A number of experts have concluded that those costs may increase over the next several decades. Thus a long-term care policy that provides a fixed amount for nursing home care—without a provision that will cover possible increases—may not cover the future costs of such care.

It's important, as well, to make certain that the policy is guaranteed to be renewable as long as you continue to pay your premiums on time. Depending on your needs and concerns, you may also want to research the question of whether the policy will offer coverage for day care programs designed for senior citizens, and coverage for some aspects of care in an assisted living facility.

The timing is important, as well. If you wait until you have a serious illness before applying for a long-term care insurance policy, you may not be able to find a company that will issue a policy for you.

Before purchasing a long-term care policy, make certain that you understand exactly what the policy offers and what the economic costs and potential benefits are. If you're not sure of the meaning of some of the terms, limitations, or exclusions discussed in the policy, request additional information from the company.

In addition, it's important to read the booklets on long-term care published by various agencies and organizations (See Appendix B). Those booklets can offer a review of the overall issues, and can also offer up-to-date information on the rules related to coverage for long-term care offered through Medicare and Medicaid.

You may also want to discuss issues related to long-term

care with a specially trained volunteer counselor. Each state has a free counseling program designed to help Medicare beneficiaries with health insurance problems. The program has a different official name in each state, but it's generally coordinated either by the state Department of Insurance, the Division on Aging, or another similar state agency. Medicare offers several publications that list the names of the relevant agencies in each state (See Appendix B). The United Seniors Health Cooperative, a private organization in Washington, D.C., can also offer information on long-term care issues.

Given the complex nature of the decision to purchase a long-term care policy, and the complicated question of when to apply for such a policy, it's essential to obtain advice from a financial planner and an attorney before making any decisions related to long-term care.

OTHER SOURCES OF COVERAGE

Although long-term care insurance policies offer important benefits for many individuals, they represent only one way to provide for long-term care. Other possible sources of benefits for long-term care include state and local government-sponsored programs, community agencies, veterans' benefit programs, Medicaid, reverse mortgages, and home equity loans.

For example, there are government-sponsored residences or apartment houses in some communities that may offer specially designed apartments as well as some basic support services for senior citizens. In some cases, rent for such apartments may be partially subsidized by the government. Because of the variety of programs available and the vast differences between those programs, it's important to review a number of assisted living facilities, retirement communities, and government-sponsored apartments or residences before making a decision. (See Appendix B for a list of booklets on this topic.)

If you have a sufficient amount of money in reserve, it may also be possible to provide for home health care or for care at a private assisted living facility without the need for insurance coverage and without the need to rely on government-sponsored programs. If you own your own house, and have sufficient equity, you may also be able to provide for long-term care in an assisted living facility or a nursing home by selling your house.

If you are planning to continue living in your house, you may be able to provide for long-term care at home through a **reverse mortgage** or a **home equity loan.** In a reverse mortgage, a bank or mortgage company makes arrangements to pay you a certain amount of money each month or, if you prefer, makes arrangements for you to draw on a pre-established line of credit. As you withdraw money, the equity that you have in your house will decrease. When your house is eventually sold, the account will be settled with the bank or mortgage company.

Determining the precise amount of available equity in your house can be somewhat complex. However, the basic idea is simple: In general, the amount of equity that's available in a house represents the difference between the current value of the house and the existing mortgage, if any. Thus, if your house is currently worth $250,000, and you owe $50,000 on your existing mortgage, your present equity is approximately $200,000.

However, the amount of money that will actually be available to you through a reverse mortgage depends on a number of factors. Those factors may include the interest rate you are paying, the closing costs involved in the mortgage, fees, the amount of equity that you have in your house, and the type of reverse mortgage you have chosen.

Check with your lender to review the different types of reverse mortgages. In addition, there are booklets that can help you understand the basic differences between various types of reverse mortgages (See Appendix B).

In a home equity loan, the individual generally receives either a single large payment or a line of credit. The amount of the payment or credit line that's available depends on a number of factors. As with a reverse mortgage, those factors include the amount of equity you have in your house, the interest rate you are paying, fees, and closing costs.

If you are considering the possibility of applying for either a reverse mortgage or a home equity loan to cover the costs of home health care, it's important to review the mortgage carefully. In addition to making certain that you understand the mortgage rules in detail, it's also important to make certain that you understand how the loan may affect your tax situation. Given the complexity of existing tax laws and the complicated economic issues involved, it's essential to discuss the possibility of a reverse mortgage or a home equity loan with family members and with an accountant and an attorney before making a decision.

There are other ways to provide for long-term care, as well. If you are a veteran, you may be able to arrange coverage for home health care or for long-term care through veterans' benefits, particularly if you have a service-connected disability. Eligible veterans may also be able to obtain prescription medications at low cost from the local Veterans' Administration clinic. (See Appendix B for a list of additional sources of information about veterans' benefits.) Depending on the area, an individual may also be able to obtain a variety of services—including housekeeping, meals, and transportation—through various local community agencies. (See Table 18 for a review of possible sources of coverage for both home-based care and long-term care in a residential facility for eligible individuals.)

If you have limited assets, you may also be able to rely on Medicaid for coverage of your medical needs under certain conditions. However, if you have significant assets, you should be aware that there are existing laws that relate to the issue of assets and Medicaid eligibility. Given the complexity of those laws, it's important to discuss the issue with an attorney before making any decisions.

Table 18
Coverage for Home-based Care and Long-term Care in a Specialized Facility

Traditional Health Insurance

Home Health Care	Day Care	Equipment
Provides only limited coverage	Not generally covered	Provides coverage if it meets the definition of medical necessity
Assisted Living	**Skilled Nursing**	**Nursing Home**
Not generally covered	Provides only limited coverage	Not generally covered

Medicare

Home Health Care	Day Care	Equipment
Provides only limited coverage	Not generally covered unless medical services are offered	Provides coverage if it meets the Medicare definition of medical necessity
Assisted Living	**Skilled Nursing**	**Nursing Home**
Not generally covered	Provides limited coverage under certain conditions	Not generally covered

Medigap Insurance

Home Health Care	Day Care	Equipment
Coverage depends on the policy	Coverage depends on the policy	Coverage depends on the policy

Table 18 (Continued)

Medigap Insurance

Assisted Living	Skilled Nursing	Nursing Home
Not generally covered	May provide limited coverage as long as the expense is viewed as eligible by Medicare	Not generally covered

Medicaid

Home Health Care	Day Care	Equipment
Coverage depends on state regulations	Coverage depends on state regulations	Provides coverage if it meets the Medicaid definition of medical necessity
Assisted Living	**Skilled Nursing**	**Nursing Home**
May provide coverage for certain types of care in states with a Medicaid waiver	Provides limited coverage	Provides coverage

Long-Term Care Insurance

Home Health Care	Day Care	Equipment
Coverage depends on the policy	Coverage depends on the policy	Not generally covered
Assisted Living	**Skilled Nursing**	**Nursing Home**
Coverage depends on the policy	Coverage depends on the policy	Coverage depends on the policy

Table 18 (Continued)

Community Agencies

Home Health Care	Day Care	Equipment
May provide meals and housekeeping	Not generally covered	Not generally covered
Assisted Living	**Skilled Nursing**	**Nursing Home**
Not generally covered	Not generally covered	Not generally covered

Veterans' Benefits

Home Health Care	Day Care	Equipment
Provides coverage	Not generally covered	Provides coverage
Assisted Living	**Skilled Nursing**	**Nursing Home**
Not generally covered	Not generally covered	Provides coverage

Reverse Mortgage or Home Equity Loan

Home Health Care	Day Care	Equipment
The amount of money available depends on equity	The amount of money available depends on equity	The amount of money available depends on equity
Assisted Living	**Skilled Nursing**	**Nursing Home**
In some cases, the loan may end if the individual moves to an assisted living facility	For short-term care; the amount of money available depends on equity	In some cases, the loan may end if the individual moves to a nursing home

Table 18 is based on the assumption that a skilled nursing facility represents a temporary treatment center—where the individual will soon be returning home—and that an assisted living facility or a nursing home represents a more permanent arrangement. In all cases where coverage may be available to eligible individuals for either home-based care or for long-term care in a specialized facility, such coverage is always limited by specific rules and regulations. In addition, claims for services or medical equipment must meet the plan's definition of medical necessity before they will be covered.

As the population ages and Americans become more aware of the importance of coverage for long-term care, government-sponsored programs and health insurance policies may be expanded to cover all such needs, or perhaps a new approach to meeting long-term care needs may be developed for all individuals. In the meantime, if you have particular concerns about the lack of coverage for long-term care under existing health insurance policies or government programs, write to your state and federal legislative representatives and let them know of those concerns.

SUMMARY

The lack of universal health insurance coverage for long-term care and the movement toward maximum independence for people with disabilities makes careful planning for long-term care essential. In addition to long-term care insurance policies, it may be possible to provide for home-based long-term care needs through a reverse mortgage or a home equity loan. In some areas, local community agencies may also offer housekeeping, meals, and transportation services. Depending on circumstances, it may also be possible to obtain coverage for long-term care through Medicaid, through local or state government-sponsored programs, or through veterans' benefits.

Given the complexity of the issues involved in planning for long-term care, it's important to research the subject carefully before making any decision. That research should include a review of booklets published by various agencies and organizations, and discussions with family members, a financial advisor, and an attorney.

Conclusion: The Future of Health Insurance in America

Since President Clinton first proposed the complete reform of the American health insurance system, national attention has been focused on health insurance-related issues with an unparalleled degree of interest. Although the Clinton proposal was never enacted into law, the discussions that it generated have made many Americans aware of the fact that the American health care system represents state-of-the-art medicine, and that individuals who are covered by comprehensive health insurance plans often receive superb care. At the same time, we've also become aware that our current system includes a number of serious problems that need to be dealt with.

First, approximately 40 million Americans are unable to derive much benefit from our system of health care because they or their families are unable to obtain health insurance coverage and cannot afford to pay for health care on their own. Unfortunately, many of the people in that group are children, including large numbers of children with disabilities.

Second, the rapid expansion of managed care has focused our attention on the need to determine the degree to which the managed care approach is effective. Will managed care result in a significant reduction in the cost of health insurance in the long run? Can it provide medical care at an appropriate level for people with a wide range of illnesses and conditions, including those with serious illnesses or disabilities? Hopefully, such questions will be answered definitively over the next few years, as research into these issues is completed.

Third, it's become clear that there is an enormous need to provide a mechanism so that individuals who lose their jobs, or who develop serious illnesses or conditions, are guaranteed the opportunity to continue health insurance coverage on a permanent basis. COBRA and the Portability and Accountability Act meet that need to some extent at this point, but they represent only a partial solution to the problem.

Fourth, we're coming to realize the importance of finding a way to improve communication between insurers and consumers. At times, statements in letters and EOBS (Explanation of Benefits Statements) from insurers are so complex and so confusing that it's almost impossible for consumers to fully understand them. That complexity makes it extremely difficult for consumers to resolve health insurance problems, and to meet insurance company requests for additional information or documentation.

Fifth, we've become aware of the need to simplify the rules that govern the Medicare program, and of the need to improve communication between Medicare and Medicare beneficiaries.

Sixth, there's growing agreement that our current paper-based health insurance claim-filing and processing system is inefficient, time-consuming, frustrating, and enormously expensive. The current system requires consumers and medical personnel to spend countless hours filling out claim forms, photocopying medical bills, and filing claims. In addition, it requires consumers to call or write to hospitals, testing centers, or doctors' offices to obtain copies of itemized bills, operative reports, doctors' letters, or other types of documentation when claim problems occur. In many cases, the current system also places the individual consumer in the middle, between the insurance company and the provider.

In contrast, an electronic claim-filing and processing system—based on the use of computers and electronic cards—could save billions of dollars in administrative costs and, at the same time, radically increase efficiency. In addition, an electronic claim-filing and processing system could completely eliminate the need for consumers to be involved in filling out claim forms, photocopying bills, and collecting documentation. Such a system could also eliminate situations in which consumers are caught in the middle—between insurance companies and providers—when routine claim-processing problems occur.

Seventh, the increasing life-span of the population and the limitations of existing government and private health insurance programs have increased our understanding of the need for universal coverage for long-term care. Currently, neither Medicare nor private health insurance policies generally provide full coverage for long-term care, and Medicaid eligibility depends on a number of factors, including income.

Eighth, although a number of important changes have been made over the last few years in the health insurance system and in the laws and regulations that govern that system, those changes represent a continuation of the piecemeal approach that has so often been followed in the past. While some of those changes have helped to solve specific problems, they have also added to the complexity of the system. The result is an intensification of the health insurance maze.

At this point, there is a desperate need for the entire American system of health insurance to be carefully reviewed. There is a need, as well, for appropriate overall changes to be made so that our system of health insurance operates more efficiently, is easier for consumers to understand, and more fully protects consumers' rights.

Finally, it's become clear that we need to make a decision as a nation about the philosophical approach we wish to adopt in terms of health insurance. Do we want a health insurance system that's based on government sponsorship and government regulation, on the free market, or on some combination of the two?

Regardless of the philosophical approach you support, the events of the last few years have made it clear that the way to effect change is for individuals to begin to participate more actively in the discussions and debates on health care and health insurance in America. There are a number of groups and organizations that currently have significant influence on those issues. However, in a democracy such as ours, no group has as much potential influence on the future of health care and health insurance in the United States as average American citizens who are united and organized around a single goal. The recent passage of the Portability and Accountability Act, the Mental Health Parity Act, the Newborns' and Mothers' Health Protection Act, and the Spina Bifida-Agent Orange Benefits Act— laws strongly supported by consumers—as well as the many new health insurance laws that have been passed on the state level, attest to that potential influence.

Given the uniqueness of the American economic and political system, and the distinctive history of America's system of health care and health insurance, it may not be possible or even wise for us to attempt to adopt some version of a health insurance plan developed in another country. However, we clearly have the intelligence, the knowledge, and the skills to develop our own unique approach to health insurance reform, without losing the medical excellence offered by our current system. I think our challenge as a nation now is to find a way to translate our ideas into reality, and to shape the future in such a way that we can ensure appropriate health insurance and health care for all Americans.

Appendix A: Ten Frequently Asked Questions about Health Insurance

QUESTION 1:

I have a lot of medical bills. I send in a number of health insurance claims each year, and I receive letters and statements from my insurance company on a regular basis. However, many of the comments and explanations on those letters and statements don't make any sense to me. Why can't I understand what the insurance company is trying to say?

ANSWER:

There may be several factors involved. First, the phrases used by insurers in letters and explanations often represent computer-generated statements, not personal responses. Second, like most fields, the health insurance industry has developed a language of its own, including a series of technical terms. Until a better system of communication is developed, you may have to learn some of the technical language of the health insurance field in order to be able to understand the messages from your insurer.

QUESTION 2:

I spend an enormous number of hours each year filling out health insurance forms, photocopying bills, maintaining records, and mailing claims to my insurer. Since I have health insurance coverage through both a primary and a secondary insurer, I have to go through that process twice. Why does there have to be so much paperwork involved in filing a health insurance claim?

ANSWER:

According to recent studies, the development of computers and electronic cards has eliminated the need for the enormous amount of paperwork that consumers need to deal with in filing health insurance claims. Replacing the current paper-based system of claim-filing and processing with a computerized, electronic system would eliminate the need for almost all of that paperwork.

An electronic system would also speed up the claim-filing process and save billions of dollars. In addition, a computerized, electronic claim-filing and processing system would eliminate the need for consumers to be involved in trying to deal with routine claim-processing problems.

QUESTION 3:

My insurance company keeps asking me for more information in regard to many of my claims. Why do they keep asking for all of that information?

ANSWER:

In order to make certain that claims are properly reimbursed, insurance companies generally require that specific documentation be included with some claims. For example, if a claim refers to medical equipment, an insurer may ask for a letter from a doctor explaining the medical need for the equipment.

If a claim is for surgery, an insurer may request an operative report—a detailed description of the surgery—from a doctor. If a claim is for a hospital stay, an insurer may request an itemized hospital bill, a detailed bill that lists the hospital charges individually. Although those requests may slow down the process, they serve to ensure that the company has made appropriate decisions in regard to claims.

The problem is that insurance companies are not often specific as to what documentation is required to allow for the processing of a particular claim to be completed. At times, that makes it extremely difficult for consumers to be certain how to respond to an insurance company request for additional information or documentation.

QUESTION 4:

My insurer recently denied a large part of a claim because it was above the UCR. That left me with a huge bill that I'm apparently responsible for paying. How does the insurance company decide on the UCR? How can I prevent similar problems in the future?

ANSWER:

The UCR (the Usual and Customary Rate) is determined on the basis of a statistical analysis of charges from medical providers in a specific geographic area. Once the UCR has been determined, it generally represents the maximum amount that an insurer will consider for reimbursement, regardless of the actual amount of the provider's bill.

The easiest way to prevent UCR-related problems in the future is to make use of the predetermination of benefits process in all expensive non-emergency situations. The predetermination of benefits process offers the consumer important information, and gives the consumer the opportunity to discuss economic issues with the provider and the insurer in advance of treatment.

QUESTION 5:

My insurer recently rejected a large claim for a hospital stay. Their explanation was that the hospitalization was not medically necessary. My doctor told me that it was essential that I enter the hospital. How can the insurer now say that the hospitalization wasn't medically necessary?

ANSWER:

Some insurance companies may use the phrase "not medically necessary" to mean that a particular treatment, test, or procedure is not covered under the terms of the policy. However, the phrase is also used to mean that more information is needed before a determination can be made as to whether the treatment, test, or procedure was medically necessary under the terms of the policy. In this case, your insurer appears to be using the phrase in the latter sense. Thus, I think that the insurer simply requires more information—perhaps including a copy of the itemized hospital bill and a letter from your doctor explaining the medical need for the hospitalization—before making a determination on whether the hospitalization is covered by the policy.

QUESTION 6:

I've just begun work with a new company. Health insurance is provided through a self-funded plan. My previous employer provided health insurance through a traditional plan. What's the difference between a self-funded plan and a traditional health insurance plan?

ANSWER:

Self-funded plans may offer benefits that are equal to—or more comprehensive than—traditional insurance plans. However, there are important differences between the two. One difference is that self-funded plans are sponsored by a corporation, a union, an association, or a state or municipal government agency, while traditional plans are generally established by insurance companies. In addition, self-funded plans are regulated under a federal law called ERISA, not under state law, in terms of benefit-related issues, and are generally exempt from state laws related to health insurance benefits.

QUESTION 7:

I have a traditional health insurance plan. I was in the hospital a few weeks ago for surgery, and I'm now receiving a number of bills from the doctors who treated me, including the surgeon and other medical specialists. I was in the hospital many years ago, and I don't remember getting more than one bill. Why am I getting so many bills? In addition, I gave the hospital all of my insurance information. I don't understand why the bills are being sent to me rather than to my insurance company.

ANSWER:

Years ago, hospitals often took care of filing bills both for the use of hospital facilities and for doctors' services. Those bills were generally sent directly to the patient's insurance company. These days, hospitals generally send only the bill for the use of hospital facilities to the insurer. Each doctor provides a separate bill for his services. Although you gave your insurance information to the hospital when you were admitted, that information may not have been shared with the doctors who provided treatment, even though they work at the hospital.

QUESTION 8:

I've been covered by Medicare for a number of years. My claims have generally been handled without major difficulty, until recently. Now, Medicare insists that I'm no longer entitled to coverage because my husband—who, in fact, died a number of years ago—is covered by a health insurance plan I've never heard of. What can I do?

ANSWER:

Medicare obtains information from a variety of sources, including other government agencies. Unfortunately, that information is not always accurate. The first step in a situation such as this is to write to your Medicare carrier (the address in on your EOMBS, the Explanation of Medicare Benefits Statement). If that does not resolve the problem, you'll need to file a Medicare appeal (the instructions are on the EOMBS). If that does not lead to a resolution of the problem, you can seek help from an organization such as the Medicare Rights Center, the United Seniors Health Cooperative, or the counseling service run by your state Department of Insurance or state Division on Aging.

QUESTION 9:

My father lives near us. He owns his own house, and he's basically healthy at this point. However, I'm worried that he may need long-term care as he gets older. He's not wealthy, and so he may not be able to afford the care he needs on his own, and we may not have the economic resources to help him. Although he's covered by Medicare, I know Medicare does not provide much coverage for long-term care. What should we do to make certain his health care needs are met in the future?

ANSWER:

There are a number of ways to provide for long-term care. A long-term care policy can provide for a variety of needs. However, such policies are not standardized. Thus, it's important to review various policies carefully to make certain that the policy that's eventually chosen will meet your father's needs in the future. Since your father owns his own house, it may also be possible for him to meet his long-term care needs through a reverse mortgage or a home equity loan. If he is a veteran with a service-connected disability, he may also be entitled to veterans' benefits. In addition, there are community agencies in most areas that provide services such as meals and house-keeping. Since providing for long-term care for an elderly person involves complex decisions that may have a number of important implications, it's essential to discuss the issues with other family members and with an accountant and an attorney before making any decision.

QUESTION 10:

My daughter has a serious disability. She's not old enough to go to school yet, but as she gets older she'll need a variety of medical equipment, including a power wheelchair. In addition, we'll need to add a wheelchair lift to our van in order to transport her more easily, and we'll need to install ramps throughout our house. We may eventually have to rebuild the bathroom, as well, to make it fully accessible. Although we have good health insurance coverage, I'm not sure that the equipment she will need will be covered by the policy. We won't be able to afford the equipment on our own. What can we do?

ANSWER:

Health insurance policies often provide coverage for power wheelchairs, but they will not usually cover related expenses such as a wheelchair-lift or home modifications. Fortunately, there are other available sources of funds for medical equipment and services for a child with a disability. For example, in many areas state agencies have funds available to purchase medical equipment for a child with a disability. Depending on the state, those funds may be provided through the state Department of Health, the Department of Insurance, the Division of Developmental Disabilities, or the Division of Vocational Rehabilitation Services. Funds may also be available through the local Independent Living Center.

When your daughter begins to attend school, the local public school district may also provide help with the purchase of medical equipment. However, that equipment must be clearly related to your daughter's educational needs, and the need for the equipment must generally be noted in her IEP. Local fraternal organizations may provide support, as well, and groups such as the Disabled Childrens' Relief Fund may provide funds for equipment that's not covered by your health insurance policy.

You may also be able to purchase used medical equipment inexpensively through your state Tech Act equipment recycling or equipment exchange program. Your local Protection and Advocacy Office or Independent Living Center should be able to help you explore those possibilities.

Appendix B: Sources of Information and Advice on Specific Health Insurance Problems

ADVOCACY GROUPS AND SUPPORT GROUPS

The Arc deals with issues related to individuals with retardation (Telephone: 1-817-261-6003).

The National Alliance for the Mentally Ill (NAMI) deals with issues related to individuals with mental or emotional illnesses (Telephone: 1-703-524-7600).

For information about other advocacy, support, and self-help groups, call the American Self-Help Clearinghouse at 1-201-625-7101.

THE ARC GROUP HEALTH INSURANCE PROGRAM

For detailed information on The Arc's group health insurance program, call Albert H. Wohlers & Company at 1-800-323-2106.

CHAMPUS/TRI-CARE

For a copy of the *CHAMPUS Handbook* write to the National Tri-Care Support Office, Benefit Services Branch, Aurora, CO 80045-6900.

To file a CHAMPUS or Tri-Care appeal, write to National Tri-Care Support Office, Office of Appeals and Hearings, Aurora, CO 80045-6900.

For specific information on CHAMPUS or Tri-Care programs, call 1-303-361-1126.

CLAIM-PROCESSING COMPANIES

For information on private medical claim-processing companies, call or write to the National Association of Claims Assistance Professionals (NACAP), 5329 S. Main St., Ste. 102, Downers Grove, IL 60515-4845 (Telephone: 1-800-660-0665; FAX: 1-800-660-9228). The local telephone directory may list additional claim-processing companies.

COBRA

For information on COBRA rules dealing with private health insurance plans, write to the Pension and Welfare Benefits Administration, United States Department of Labor, N5619, 200 Constitution Ave. NW, Washington, DC 20210, or call 1-202-219-8776.

For information on COBRA rules dealing with health insurance plans sponsored by a state or municipal government agency, write to Department of Health and Human Services, Division of Cost Allocation, COBRA, Room 1067, Cohen Bldg., 330 Independence Ave. SW, Washington, DC 20210.

DISABILITIES

The following booklets are available from The Arc, a national organization on mental retardation

- "Appealing a Social Security Disability Benefits Decision" (Booklet 101-44);
- "Social Security and SSI Benefits for Children with Disabilities" (Booklet 101-36).

For current prices and for further information, write to Publications, The Arc, National Headquarters, P.O. Box 1047,

Arlington, TX 76004 (Telephone: 1-817-261-6003; TTY: 1-817-277-0553).

The *EPSDT Handbook*, a technical manual that describes the program rules for the Early Periodic Screening, Diagnosis, and Treatment Program, is available from the National Health Law Program for $30 (Telephone: 1-310-204-6010).

Exceptional Parent Magazine, a monthly magazine devoted to the needs of parents of children with disabilities, can be ordered by calling 1-800-247-8080.

The following organizations offer help and advice with specific problems related to Medicaid and disability issues

- Bazelon Center for Mental Health Law deals with legal issues related to mental health (Telephone: 1-202-467-5730);
- Children's Defense Fund deals with legal issues related to children with disabilities (In the New York area, call 1-212-233-4000; outside New York, call 1-202-628-8787);
- Disability Law Centers deal with disability-related legal and health insurance issues (In New York City, contact Disability Law Center at New York Lawyers for the Public Interest, 1-212-727-2270; outside New York, contact the Disability Rights Education and Defense Fund, 1-800-466-4232);
- Legal Services deals with legal issues related to health insurance problems involving children or adults who have limited economic resources (Call the National Legal Aid and Defender Association at 1-202-452-0620 or the local Bar Association for the telephone number of the nearest office);
- Protection and Advocacy Service deals with Medicaid problems related to children with disabilities (Call the local Bar Association for the number of the nearest office).

The Disabled Children's Relief Fund provides grants to help purchase medical equipment for children with disabilities (Write to Disabled Children's Relief Fund, 402 Pennsylvania Ave, Freeport, NY 11520, or call 1-516-377-1605; Fax: 1-516-377-3978).

Telephone Pioneers helps with disability-related engineering projects and modifications (Telephone: 1-303-571-9270).

Tech Act programs provide information on used medical equipment (Call RESNA—the Rehabilitation Engineering and Assistive Technology Society of North America—for information on state Tech Act programs; telephone: 1-703-524-6686).

For information on the "Prescription Drug Patient Assistance Program" write to the Pharmaceutical Research and Manufacturers of America, 1100 Fifteenth Street NW, Washington, D.C. 20005. Ask for a free copy of the "1997 Directory of Prescription Drug Patient Assistance Programs."

ELECTRONIC CLAIM-PROCESSING

For a copy of the study by Thomas Edison College and the New Jersey Institute of Technology on the development of a computerized, electronic claim-filing and processing system write to Thomas Edison State College, 101 West State St., Trenton, NJ 08680-1176 (Attn: Mark Gordon); include a check for $30.

ERISA

For information on ERISA regulations, write to the Pension and Welfare Benefits Administration, United States Department of Labor, N 5619, 200 Constitution Ave. NW, Washington, DC 20210, or call 1-202-219-8776.

HEALTH MAINTENANCE ORGANIZATIONS

For information on the accreditation of a specific HMO, write to the National Committee for Quality Assurance, 2000 L St. NW, Ste. 500, Washington, DC 20036 (Internet site: http://www.ncqa.org; telephone: 1-202-955-3500; Fax: 1-202-955-3599).

For a copy of the *Health Plan Guide*, a publication based on a survey of federal employees concerning HMOs, write to the

Center for the Study of Services, 733 15th St. NW, Washington, DC 20005.

To request help with a specific health insurance problem involving an HMO—where appeals to the HMO itself and to state agencies have been unsuccessful—write to either the National Committee for Quality Assurance, 2000 L St. NW, Ste. 500, Washington, DC 20036, or to the American Association of Health Plans, Communications Department, 20th St. NW, Ste. 600, Washington, DC 20036.

LONG-TERM CARE

The following booklets are available from the United Seniors Health Cooperative

- "Home Care for Older People: A Consumer's Guide;"
- "Long-Term Care: A Dollars and Sense Guide;"
- "Long-Term Care Insurance: A Professional's Guide to Selecting Policies;"
- "Private Long-Term Care Insurance: To Buy or Not to Buy?"

For current prices and further information, write to United Seniors Health Cooperative, 1331 H St. NW, # 500, Washington, DC 20005-4706 (Telephone: 1-202-393-6222; Fax: 1-202-783-0588).

Medicare's *Guide to Health Insurance for People with Medicare* and the *Medicare Handbook* list state agencies that offer free counseling programs for Medicare beneficiaries in terms of Medicare, Medigap, and long-term care. Those booklets should be available from the local Social Security Office.

"Reverse Mortgage Locator" ($1; include a self-addressed, stamped, business size envelope)—a list of lenders who offer reverse mortgages in each state—and *Your New Retirement Nest Egg: A Consumer Guide to the New Reverse Mortgages* ($24.95, plus $4.50 shipping and handling) are available from the National Center for Home Equity Conversion, 7373 147 St. W., Apple Valley, MN 55124.

MEDICARE

The following booklets are available from the Medicare Rights Center

- "How To Avoid Overpaying Your Doctor under Medicare: Part B" and "Your Doctor's Bills" (an explanation of the rules regarding assignment, limiting charges, and other related issues);
- "How to Receive Medicare Home Benefits" (a discussion of the rules relating to Medicare coverage for home care);
- "Medicare and Employer Health Insurance: How They Work Together" (a discussion of the question of how to determine whether Medicare is primary or secondary in situations in which a Medicare beneficiary's spouse is covered by an employer-sponsored group health insurance plan);
- "Medicare Basics—Your Medicare Health Insurance Options" (an overview of the Medicare system);
- "Medicare HMOs" (a discussion of issues related to the question of whether to join a Medicare HMO or to continue with the traditional Medicare plan);
- "Medicare Supplemental Insurance" (an outline of the standardized Medigap plans and a discussion of related issues);
- "Your Appeal Rights Under Medicare: Part B" (an explanation of the Medicare appeals system in regard to outpatient claims);
- "QMB and SLMB: Programs for Low-Income Beneficiaries" (an explanation of the federal Qualified Medicare Beneficiary program and the Selected Low-Income Medicare Beneficiary program).

The *Medicare Survival Kit* includes all of these booklets, as well as additional information on Medicare and Medigap policies. Other booklets are published from time to time. For a list of current prices and for further information, write to Medicare Rights Center, 1460 Broadway, 8th Floor, New York, NY 10036 (Attn: John Miller), or call 1-212-869-3850.

The following booklets are available from the United Seniors Health Cooperative

- "Medicare HMOs: Some Tips for Consumers" (a review of rules related to Medicare HMOs);
- "Medicare, Medigap, and Managed Care: Consumer Update" (an overview of Medicare, Medigap, and managed care programs);
- "Managing Your Health Care Finances: Getting the Most Out of Medicare and Medigap Insurance" (a review of current rules for Medicare and Medigap policies);
- *United Seniors Health Report Newsletter*, published five times a year (reviews recent changes in Medicare and Medicare-related programs).

Other booklets are published from time to time. For current prices and information, write to United Seniors Health Cooperative, 1331 H St. NW, # 500, Washington, DC 20005-4706 (Telephone: 1-202-393-6222; Fax: 1-202-783-0588).

The Medicare Handbook, which lists many of the current Medicare rules, is available from your local Social Security Office.

The following organizations and agencies offer help with specific problems related to Medicare and Medigap policies

- Medicare Inspector-General (issues related to Medicare fraud; to report possible Medicare fraud call or write Health and Human Services, Office of the Inspector-General, P.O. Box 17303, Baltimore, MD 21203-7303; Telephone: 1-800-368-5779);
- Medicare Rights Center (Telephone: 1-212-869-3850);
- State-sponsored counseling programs, operated by trained volunteers (the programs have different official names in each of the states, but are generally supervised by the state Department of Insurance or the Division on Aging);
- United Seniors Health Cooperative (Telephone: 1-202-393-6222; Fax: 1-202-783-0588).

In addition, if you have access to a computer you can find a variety of information on Medicare deductibles, co-insurance, and related issues on Medicare's home page. The address is http://www.HCFA.gov.

VETERANS' BENEFITS

For information on veterans' benefits related to home health care, coverage for prescription medications, or long-term care, call your local Veterans' Administration office, or call the Paralyzed Veterans' of America at 1-202-872-1300 (in the New York area, call the Eastern Paralyzed Veterans' Association at 1-718-803-EPVA).

Glossary

Assisted Living Facility. A residential facility designed to provide a range of supportive services—including meals, housekeeping, and medical services—for senior citizens.

Balance Bill. The difference between the provider's bill and the amount of reimbursement offered by the insurance company.

Basic Benefits. The provision in a traditional health insurance policy that provides coverage for specific medical tests, ambulance service, and other services.

CHAMPUS (Civilian Health and Medical Program of the Uniformed Services). A health benefits system for eligible dependents of armed services personnel and for eligible retired armed services personnel.

Claim Appeal. A request that an insurer review a specific claim and the level of reimbursement.

COBRA (Congressional Omnibus Budget Reconciliation Act). A set of federal regulations designed to allow for a temporary continuation of health insurance benefits for eligible individuals.

Co-insurance. The percentage of a medical bill that an individual is obligated to pay, according to the policy.

Conversion Option. A provision contained in some group health insurance plans that permits a person to convert a group policy to an individual policy, thus allowing for additional benefits when the lifetime benefit maximum has been reached.

Coordination-of-Benefits. A system for providing secondary benefits in a situation in which an individual is covered under more than one health insurance plan.

Co-payment. *See* Co-insurance.

Day Care Program. A specialized, non-residential program for senior citizens that offers a range of recreational and medical services.

Documentation. The paperwork that insurers generally require before processing a claim; it may include a letter of medical necessity, an operative report, or an itemized hospital bill.

Durable Medical Equipment. Equipment such as a manual or power wheelchair, braces, or a walker.

Electronic Claim-filing System. A system of health insurance claim-filing and processing through the use of computers and electronic cards.

EOBS (Explanation of Benefits Statement). The statement sent by an insurer to a consumer, listing charges, dates of service, the amount of reimbursement, and an explanation of the insurer's determination of that amount.

EOMBS (Explanation of Medicare Benefits Statement). A statement from Medicare that includes the name of the provider, the dates of service, the Medicare allowable amount, and other related information.

Equipment Exchange or Recycling Program. A system for selling or buying used durable medical equipment, established through the various Tech Act programs.

ERISA (Employee Retirement Income Security Act). A federal law that regulates the operation of self-funded plans.

Family Coverage. Coverage for dependents.

Family Deductible. A provision that allows an insurer to assume that the yearly individual deductible has been met for all family members once several family members have met the deductible.

Fee-for-Service Plan. *See* Traditional Plan.

Gatekeeper. *See* Primary Care Physician.

Group Plan. A health insurance plan provided through a group such as a corporation or a business.

HCFA (Health Care Financing Administration). The federal agency responsible for regulating Medicare.

Home Equity Loan. A loan from a bank or mortgage company based on the equity in a house; the loan can be used to provide for long-term health care or for health insurance needs.

Hospital Benefits (Inpatient). Benefits for an overnight stay in a hospital; the benefits include coverage for room, food, and nursing care.

Hospital Benefits (Outpatient). Benefits for treatment in a hospital emergency room or a hospital same-day surgery facility, or for tests performed in a hospital on an outpatient basis; claims may be covered under major medical.

HMO (Health Maintenance Organization). A managed care plan that has a network of doctors, hospitals, and testing centers, and provisions such as a requirement for pre-authorization prior to specific treatments, tests, or services.

IEP. *See* Individualized Education Program.

Indemnity Plan. *See* Traditional Plan.

Individual Policy. A health insurance policy purchased individually rather than through a group.

Individualized Education Program (IEP). A plan filed with the local school district that summarizes specific educational goals for a child with a disability.

Legal Services. An agency located in each state that provides help with legal problems—including help with health insurance issues—for eligible individuals.

Letter of Medical Necessity. A letter from a doctor explaining the medical need for a particular treatment or procedure.

Lifetime Benefit Maximum. The maximum amount of reimbursement that an insurance policy will provide for specific benefits during a person's lifetime.

Long-term Care Insurance. An insurance policy designed to provide coverage for long-term care expenses that are not generally covered either by individual or group health insurance plans or by Medicare.

Major Medical Benefits. The portion of a health insurance plan that provides coverage for treatment by a doctor, for same-day surgery, and for medical tests that are not covered under basic benefits.

Managed Care Organization (MCO). *See* Managed Care Plan.

Managed Care Plan. A health plan that has a network of doctors, hospitals, and testing centers, and provisions such as a requirement for pre-authorization prior to specific treatments, tests, or services; includes HMOs and PPOs.

Master Contract. A group health insurance agreement between an employer and an insurer.

MCO. *See* Managed Care Plan.

Medicaid. A health insurance program sponsored jointly by the federal and state governments, designed to provide insurance for people whose income is below the poverty line and for many children with disabilities.

Medicaid EPSDT Program. A Medicaid program that may provide coverage for certain types of medical problems that are identified during an EPSDT screening of a child with a disability.

Medicaid HMO. An HMO designed specifically for Medicaid recipients.

Medicaid Waiver. An agreement to exempt a state from a particular set of federal Medicaid regulations; a specific waiver may relate to the way in which services are provided or to eligibility for specific services.

Medicare. A health insurance program sponsored by the federal government, designed to provide insurance for senior citizens and for some children and adults with disabilities.

Medicare Allowable Amount. The charge allowed under Medicare rules for a specific service, test, or procedure.

Medicare Beneficiaries Incentive Program. A program designed to encourage Medicare beneficiaries to report possible cases of fraud.

Medicare HMO. An HMO designed specifically for Medicare beneficiaries.

Medicare Limiting Charge. The maximum percentage above the allowable amount that a nonparticipating provider can generally charge a Medicare beneficiary.

Medicare Nonparticipating Provider. A provider that does not accept the Medicare allowable amount as the fee.

Medicare Participating Provider. A provider that accepts the Medicare allowable amount as the fee.

Medigap Policy. A policy designed to help Medicare beneficiaries pay for Medicare deductible and co-insurance amounts, and for other specific services.

Mental and Emotional Illness Provision. A provision in a health insurance plan that includes coverage for the treatment of depression, anxiety, schizophrenia, bipolar disorder, and similar illnesses or conditions.

Mental Health Parity Act. A federal law passed in October of 1996 that prohibits insurers and self-funded plans that offer coverage for the treatment of mental illnesses from establishing lower yearly or lifetime maximums for reimbursement for the treatment of mental illnesses than for the treatment of physical illnesses. A number of states have also passed laws that deal with the issue of mental health parity.

Newborns' and Mothers' Health Protection Act. A federal law passed in the fall of 1996 that requires all insurance policies and self-funded plans that offer coverage for childbirth to provide benefits for a full 48 hours of hospital care in relation to childbirth and 96 hours of hospital care in relation to a Caesarean delivery.

Not Medically Necessary. A term used by insurers to mean either that additional documentation is required before the insurer can determine whether a treatment is medically necessary, or that a decision has been made that a treatment is not covered under the terms of the policy.

Nursing Home. A residential facility designed to provide personal care for senior citizens with severe chronic conditions or disabilities.

Operative Report. A detailed description of an operation, usually written by the physician who performed the surgery.

Outpatient Treatment for Mental Illness. Therapy sessions with a psychologist, psychiatrist, or other mental health professional to treat mental or emotional illnesses.

Parity. Equality of benefits in terms of coverage for the treatment of mental and physical illnesses or conditions.

Participating Provider. A doctor, hospital, or testing center that is part of a plan network.

Percentile. The level of an array of charges at which reimbursement will generally be provided by an insurer.

Plan Administrator. An insurance company or other agency that administers a self-funded plan; benefit-related decisions are generally made on the basis of rules set by the plan sponsor rather than by the insurer.

Plan Sponsor. A corporation, union, association, or state or municipal government agency that has established a self-funded plan.

Point-of-Service (POS) Option. An option in a managed care plan that provides reimbursement for non-network providers, though often at a lower level.

Portability and Accountability Act. A federal law passed in 1996 that allows consumers to transfer to a new health insurance plan without exclusions for pre-existing conditions under certain conditions, provides for the establishment of Medical Savings Accounts, and contains a series of provisions related to Medicare, Medicaid, and group health insurance plans.

PPO (Preferred Provider Organization). A managed care plan in which a participant may use either network providers or non-network providers; reimbursement is generally higher if network providers are used.

Pre-authorization. The requirement that a plan participant generally receive approval before entering a hospital or before arranging for expensive medical tests or services.

Predetermination of Benefits. A request that an insurer provide information prior to treatment about the amount of reimbursement that may be available for a particular procedure under the terms of the insurance policy.

Preventive Care. Medical care related to the prevention of illnesses rather than to their treatment; it may include vaccinations, screening tests, and routine yearly physicals.

Primary Care Physician. A provider in a managed care plan who is responsible for coordinating care and for approving medical tests or consultations with a specialist.

Procedure Code. A code given to a specific medical treatment, test, or procedure; it is used by insurers in processing claims.

Provider (Provider of Service). A doctor, hospital, or testing center that provides treatment or medical services.

Qualified Medicare Beneficiary Program. A program designed to help eligible Medicare beneficiaries pay for Medicare deductibles and other related expenses.

Reinsurance Program. A program that may be used by some self-funded plans to cover claims beyond a predetermined amount.

RESNA (Rehabilitation Engineering and Assistive Technology Society of North America). The agency that serves as the technical consultant for the Tech Act programs.

Reverse Mortgage. A mortgage that provides an individual home owner with monthly payments or a line of credit from a bank or mortgage company based on the equity in a house; the money may be used to provide for long-term health care or health insurance needs.

Rider. A provision added to a health insurance policy that may provide benefits for specific items that are not covered under the standard policy, including eyeglasses, hearing aids, or other medical services or equipment.

Secondary Benefits. *See* Coordination-of-Benefits.

Selected Low-Income Medicare Beneficiary Program. A program designed to help eligible Medicare beneficiaries pay for Medicare deductibles.

Self-funded Plan. A health benefit plan organized by a corporation for its employees, by a union or an association for its members, or by a state or municipal government agency.

Skilled Nursing Facility. A residential facility designed to provide skilled nursing care, often following a hospital stay.

Spina Bifida-Agent Orange Benefits Act. A federal law that was passed in 1996 that provides benefits for children and adults with spina bifida whose biological parents were exposed to Agent Orange during the Vietnam conflict.

Tech Act Programs. Programs established under the 1988 federal Technology-Related Assistance for Individuals with Disabilities Act.

Traditional Plan. A health insurance plan that allows a participant to choose any medical provider; following treatment, the participant pays the bill and sends it to the insurer for reimbursement.

Tri-Care Extra. A PPO option within the CHAMPUS program, part of the standard CHAMPUS plan.

Tri-Care Prime. A managed care option within the CHAMPUS program.

Tri-Care Standard. The traditional CHAMPUS program.

TTY. A teletype writer; designed to enable the deaf to communicate by telephone.

UCR (Usual and Customary Rate). The maximum amount that an insurer will generally consider for reimbursement; it is usually determined by a statistical analysis of claims for a particular procedure in a specific geographic area.

Yearly Co-payment Maximum. The maximum amount that an individual has to pay each year before the insurer will provide reimbursement for covered major medical claims at the 100% rate.

Yearly Individual Deductible. The amount an individual needs to pay each year before the insurer will generally begin to pay major medical claims.

Index

About the Author

RICHARD EPSTEIN writes a nationally syndicated newspaper column, "Insurance TroubleShooter," as well as a health insurance column for *Exceptional Parent Magazine*. With a BA degree from Brooklyn College, a masters from the New School for Social Research, and additional post-graduate work at the New School and at Columbia University, Epstein began researching the health insurance maze 15 years ago, after his spinal arthritis became so severe that he required an electric wheelchair for mobility. He found that many of the rules that insurance companies followed seemed illogical and, at times, almost incomprehensible.